Advance Praise for
DANGEROUS MISINFORMATION

"Dr. Mary Talley Bowden was right all along."

—**Tucker Carlson**, Author and Political Commentator

"When people of integrity are not believed, they let time prove them right."

—**John Rich**, Grammy-Nominated Artist

"Dr. Bowden, you're my spirit animal."

—**Shelley Luther**, State Representative Texas House District 62

"Crisis doesn't build character, it reveals it. Dr. Mary Talley Bowden is my doctor, and my friend. I deeply admire her courage during the insanity of COVID, and her commitment to ensuring that craziness never happens again. She risked it all to save our freedom."

—**Michael Berry**, Host of *The Michael Berry Show*

DANGEROUS MISINFORMATION

DANGEROUS MISINFORMATION

THE **VIRUS**, THE **TREATMENTS**, AND THE **LIES**

MARY TALLEY BOWDEN, MD

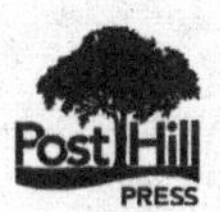

A POST HILL PRESS BOOK

Dangerous Misinformation:
The Virus, the Treatments, and the Lies

ISBN: 979-8-89565-465-1
ISBN (eBook): 979-8-89565-466-8

Cover design by Cody Corcoran

This book contains advice and information relating to health care. It should be used to supplement rather than replace the advice of your doctor or another trained health professional. You are advised to consult your health professional with regard to matters related to your health, and in particular regarding matters that may require diagnosis or medical attention. All efforts have been made to assure the accuracy of the information in this book as of the date of publication. The publisher and the author disclaim liability for any medical outcomes that may occur as a result of applying the methods suggested in this book.

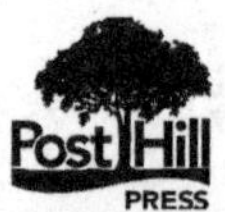

Post Hill Press
New York • Nashville
posthillpress.com

Published in the United States of America
1 2 3 4 5 6 7 8 9 10

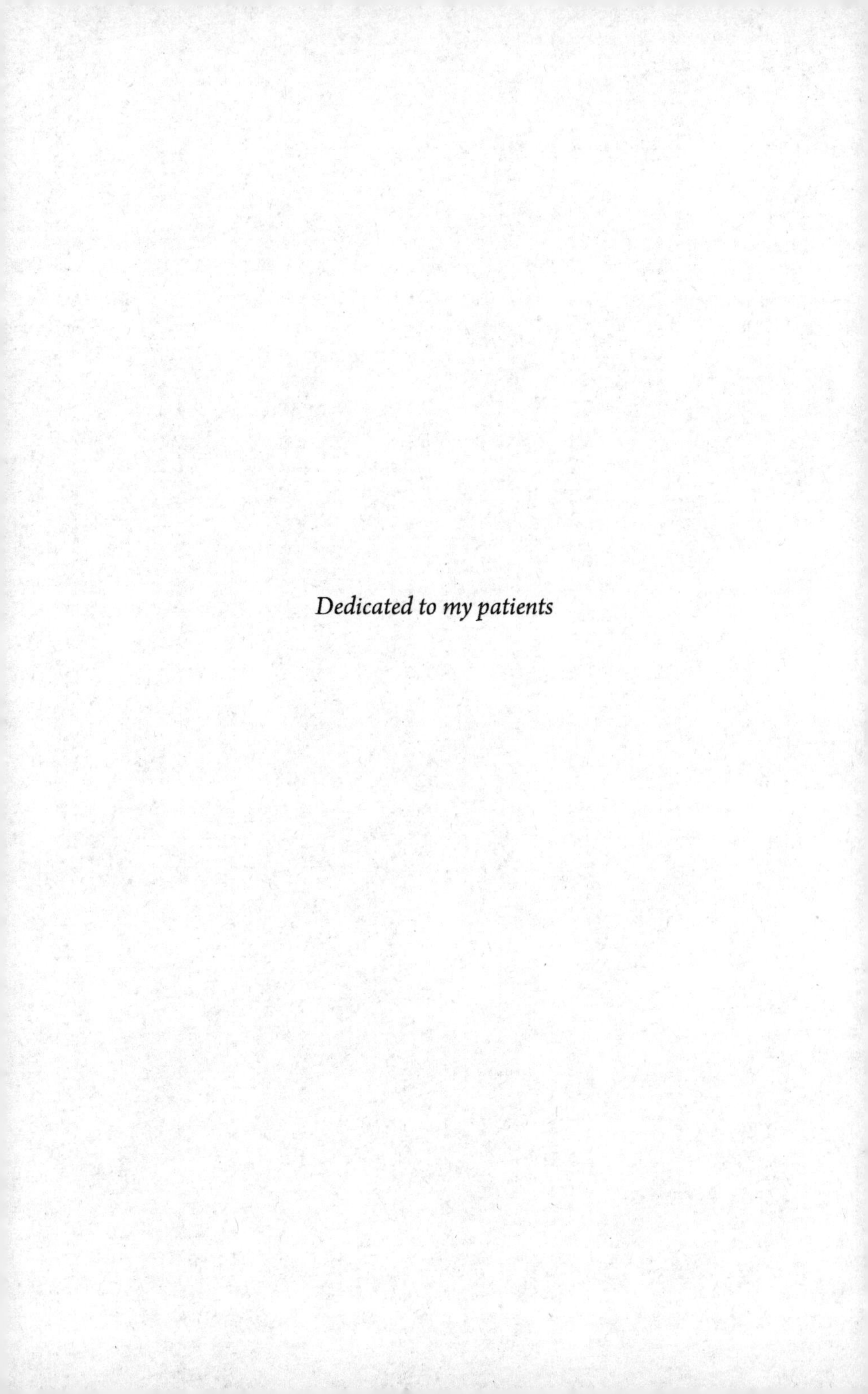

Dedicated to my patients

Contents

Intro

COVID was a highly predictable disease, easy to diagnose without a test, and because it was virtually the only illness I treated for two years, I quickly mastered it. The disease started like any other viral illness, and most recovered with minimal or no treatment, but in the small percentage who struggled, Day Eight was a turning point. By the eighth day of symptoms, patients either began the road to recovery or started to spiral down the drain.

With COVID's predictable time course, I learned the importance of early interventions to thwart possible death. In my hands, proper treatment before Day Eight guaranteed survival. After Day Eight, a subset of patients, typically those with multiple comorbid conditions who did not receive early treatment, markedly worsened as a tidal wave of inflammation gripped their bodies. I gained extensive experience preventing patients from getting to this point and a more limited, but highly rewarding, experience saving patients who came to me late and under other circumstances would have likely died in the hospital.

I successfully treated over six thousand COVID patients; I've never treated this many patients with one disease in my career and likely never will again. Nonetheless, the impact I made was minimal in the grand scheme of a worldwide pandemic. Were it not for social media, I would have likely been left alone. But when I made the mistake of sharing my findings publicly, international media branded me as "dangerous," and my life changed in ways I'd never imagined.

Prior to the pandemic, medicine as a profession enjoyed a sterling reputation. Hospitals were regarded as safe havens where well-meaning physicians and nurses used every power at their disposal to save lives. Doctors welcomed sick patients, and pharmacists filled their prescriptions, barring any legitimate safety concerns. The seeds of corruption were present but well hidden. It took the largest public health event of our time for them to sprout.

Fear drives people to embrace the arms of authority, and during the pandemic, the arms of authority returned the embrace and squeezed hard. COVID killed a lot of people unnecessarily, and in the process, uncovered massive failures in our public health system. Like the "emperor with no clothes," our government leaders commanded, "Trust the experts," while delivering a chaotic and flawed response shrouded in a guise of certainty. Doctors and nurses were neutered, as bureaucrats meant to control purse strings morphed into bureaucrats controlling patient care.

The pandemic should have been a wake-up call, but even with a new administration at the helm, few are willing to talk about the one issue that directly impacted every single American. I write this memoir as one of the few physicians who stood up to and tried to take down Goliath. It turns out the forces I faced are larger and stronger than Goliath, but the journey has been meaningful.

CHAPTER 1

The Backstory

In March of 2020, I stumbled into a new realm of medicine and a new realm of life. As rumors abounded of a virulent infection spreading quickly from China, many of my patients agonized whether or not to cancel their planned spring break vacations. My first patient was mild but memorable. Family friends brought in their teenage daughter with stubborn bronchitis—she had just returned from a school trip to China. None of us suspected COVID. We only realized in retrospect.

Spring break is normally a slow week for doctors, but this one was uniquely busy. I had heard a bit about the new virus, but like most things that appear in the news, I thought the odds of seeing it firsthand were low. I had a quiet solo practice, having only opened it six months prior. The majority of patients who came in that week had bronchitis, and as an ear, nose, and throat (ENT) specialist, I was seeing what I was accustomed to seeing.

The nose is the body's first line of defense against most respiratory pathogens; as organs go, it's my favorite and my area of expertise. I've examined thousands, and with a peek, I can distinguish between allergies and infection. I can generally tell when someone has a viral versus a bacterial infection. Though many of my ENT colleagues have become full-time surgeons, I enjoy the nonsurgical side of my specialty and have a reputation for being conservative in taking patients to the operating room. My approach is unconventional in that I don't rush—I dedicate forty-five minutes of time for new patients. I enjoy the challenge of seeing the ones other doctors can't fix, and I approach each problem like a detective trying to solve a mystery, valuing a thorough history and physical exam over a slew of tests. I approached COVID as any other respiratory tract infection I was used to treating. I had no reservations in helping my patients when they sought help from me.

When the pandemic started, I had just returned to work after a prolonged nonacademic sabbatical. In my thirties, I gave birth to four boys in five years and put my career on hold. Four babies in five years was not part of the plan when I chose medicine as a career—in fact, when we got married, my husband and I didn't plan on even having kids. I loved being a doctor, and having spent most of my teenage years babysitting a family of four boys, I feared motherhood would be much harder than practicing medicine. But with the help of time, the memories of babysitting faded, and thoughts of becoming a mother took over. When I was thirty-four, I gave birth to my first son.

Pregnancy forces most women into the throes of our medical system. Up until that time, I was administering treatment, not receiving it. Because I know what's on the other side of the curtain, I will never fully understand what it's like to be a patient, but spending nearly five straight years in my obstetrician's office, I gained a healthy appreciation for what most patients go through.

Texas has more hospitals than any other state, and Houston is home to the largest medical center in the world, the Texas Medical

Center. Similar to the Vegas Strip with large sums of money flowing through varied institutions, hundreds of medical offices and hospitals line Fannin Street, a bustling, one-way corridor teeming with ambulances and professionals in white coats. Navigating the medical center is a daunting task. After locating the correct hospital, the next obstacle is its multi-story parking garage. I budgeted twenty dollars and an extra thirty minutes to park and make the trek from the garage to the clinic, a journey involving two crowded elevator rides and a half-mile walk.

Once I finally reached my obstetrician's office, I approached the frosted glass window, filled out a form, wordlessly nudged it to the person on the other side of the glass, and found a seat. The form never changed, and I must have filled it out a hundred times by the time all four of my children were born. The receptionists came and went, but they all had the same curt demeanor, rarely making eye contact or calling me by name.

I was considered and usually treated as a VIP, given that I was a physician. But I still waited. And I never knew how long that wait would be. I sometimes saw my doctor, but I often saw his nurse practitioner. My doctor was wonderful and delivered all four of my children—I was lucky. But visiting his office wrecked my day, and given how often I was there, I grew weary of it.

I continued to work after my first two children were born, but I never felt at ease leaving them with a nanny. With a miscarriage in between, my second son was born sixteen months after the first. The boys were high energy and exhausting, but I adored them and missed them and worried about them when I was gone. I envied the women I knew who went back to work without a hint of anxiety. My husband worked long hours and traveled extensively. Neither of us had family in town and juggling it all became untenable.

Midway through my third pregnancy, I decided to take a year off. At that time, I was working with two other ENTs in a small clinic situated next to Memorial Hermann Northwest Hospital, about five miles north of the Texas Medical Center. My employer, Dr. Kyle McCutcheon, was ten years my senior and allowed me plenty of autonomy. The day I started, fresh out of training, he left for a month of vacation—trial by fire but a great test to build my confidence. Dr. Alasdair Gilchrist, the other ENT, was a semi-retired Brit who focused on treating patients with vertigo. Hailing from an earlier era of medicine, he shared tales of practicing in the rural English countryside, where doctors used now unconventional drugs, such as heroin, to speed up childbirth when labor was prolonged.

I enjoyed the camaraderie in our practice as well as that with many of the physicians who shared privileges at the adjoining hospital. I had been there for seven years and was content and reluctant to leave. I half joked to Dr. McCutcheon that I was choosing between continuing to work and getting a divorce; he graciously blessed my departure without animosity. I promised I'd be back in a year if he still needed me.

Staying home to be a full-time mom was the right decision—divorce was averted, at least temporarily—but the one-year sabbatical didn't turn out quite as I had expected. Soon after our third child was born, we conceived again, and at the age of forty, I gave birth to our fourth son. Our oldest was only five years old at the time. Coinciding with his birth, my husband received a major promotion requiring more travel, and my plans to return to medicine were put on indefinite hold.

I embraced my role as a full-time mother and decided to not worry about the career I set aside. I had my hands full and viewed motherhood as my second career. I kept my medical license up-to-date as a safeguard but did not dwell on whether or not I would return to work. Keeping four young boys fed, bathed, clothed, and basically alive was a monumental task. The hardships of medical training prepared me for the work with the rewards being much greater. I gained valuable experience on the patient side of things, with countless visits to the pediatrician and a few to the hospital. My knowledge in examining ears paid off and saved me from more trips to the pediatrician's office than most mothers, but after a few years, I became more mom than doctor and wasn't sure I would ever go back to practicing medicine.

As the boys got older, more self-sufficient and settled into school, medicine started tugging my sleeve. I brushed it aside at first, but the tug grew stronger. I had morphed into a full-time mother and wasn't confident I would remember how to be a doctor, much less a surgeon. I didn't need to work—my husband was supporting us on his income—so to satisfy the tug, I thought I'd look at doing something in health sciences, but not necessarily medicine.

I took a class in epidemiology at the McGovern Medical School at UTHealth Houston to get a taste of nonclinical medicine, which led me to apply to the PhD translational biology and microbiology programs at Baylor Graduate School of Biomedical Sciences. The idea to go to graduate school started after applications were due, but I tried anyway, hoping to pick up an unfilled position. I crammed for the GRE (Graduate Record Examinations—I can't remember my score and was unable to find it online, but remember feeling humbled), tracked down and obtained a recommendation from one of my (retired) mentors at Stanford University, Dr. Richard Goode, and prepared a personal statement. I was a forty-three-year-old mother of four who last touched academics fifteen years earlier; not surprisingly, I didn't get accepted. It's a rejection I am now extremely grateful for and have wondered if I narrowly missed working under the infamous vaccine crusader and Baylor professor Dr. Peter Hotez.

Friends had other suggestions. One told me she wished her ENT would irrigate and suction out her sinuses and suggested I start a sinus spa. I ran this idea by my mentor, Dr. Goode, a prolific inventor with an ear tube in his name (the Goode T-tube). He embraced the idea and related an interesting story about cocaine packs in the nose:

> Mary Talley,
>
> Don't forget that your idea might be best protected by copyright or trademark. SinuSpa has a nice ring to it. I wonder if you just need a vibrating chair for relaxation and a Grossan type sinus nebulizer capable of delivering heated medications and mist. My father-in-law, a Los Angeles school principal, loved his sinus treatments. Dark room, music, comfortable chair and packs in nose for 30 minutes. Afterwards he felt great for hours. Of course it was the 10% cocaine packs that he loved (he did not know what was on them but I did). Don't think you can get away with that today ???????
>
> Dick Goode

While visiting my in-laws in western Massachusetts one Christmas, I developed a painful sinus infection in my maxillary sinus (the cheek sinus). I called in antibiotics for myself, but the pharmacist refused to fill the prescription—perhaps because I was self-prescribing and from a different state; I don't recall the reason. The pressure became intense, so I sat in the bathroom with the shower blasting, inhaling the steam, and placed a wet, hot towel over the affected sinus. I tapped the skin over my sinus hoping to dislodge something, increasing the force to the point of practically punching myself in the face. It took several minutes, but at last, I felt a gush of fluid run down the back of my throat as my sinus became unclogged, and I experienced instant relief. I realized antibiotics might not be the only way to treat a sinus infection and thought harder about the sinus spa idea.

A mom friend of mine was an internist who worked in a concierge practice. She also had four kids and a very busy husband but managed to make it look easy. Her hours were flexible, and because she didn't take insurance, she had fewer patients. Her patients texted her, and she made house calls. I was intrigued. As a specialist, it would not have made sense for me to set up a concierge practice. The problems an ENT treats typically don't require multiple visits over a lifetime and are often handled in a short-term or sporadic fashion. But I liked the concept of lower volume, higher quality care and eliminating insurance companies from the equation. In my previous job, I had hated the stranglehold insurance companies had over patient care. I only knew of two ways to practice ENT—private group practice or academics—and both entailed working for other people and taking insurance. I wasn't sure anyone would hire me after my prolonged sabbatical, and with four kids, I needed more autonomy and flexibility than most employers would be willing to tolerate. If I tried to do the traditional model on my own (taking insurance), I would have no negotiating power with insurance companies. Solo practices are mostly a thing of the past for this reason, and I knew I didn't want to feel pressured to see a high volume of patients to keep afloat.

I had become active in an online chat group of ENTs run by the American Academy of Otolaryngology and found it an invaluable resource not only for clinical information but also for learning about the business side of medicine. After seeing what my internist friend was doing, I floated the idea of starting a cash-only, insurance-free, solo ENT practice. This direct pay model cuts out the middleman to allow doctors to spend more time with their patients and less time and resources dealing with third parties such as insurance companies and the government. Price transparency and easy access are advantages of the direct pay model. I planned on listing my prices and allowing patients to book their appointments through my website. After their appointment, patients would receive a detailed invoice and submit their own claim to their insurance company for reimbursement. I wasn't sure how I'd work out the surgery component without taking insurance, but consistent with my personality, I figured I could find a way.

The response from my colleagues was abundant and discouraging—the overwhelming response was I'd never survive. Fortunately, one brave soul was years ahead of me, setting up a cash-only practice in rural Louisiana for dizzy patients. He was kind enough to talk to me and encouraged me to take the risk, telling me if I offered something unique, patients would be willing to pay out-of-pocket.

Preparing to start the new practice took two years of researching and networking and building my confidence. I took medical and surgical courses to refresh my skills—thankfully operating was like riding a bike and the skills came back much more easily than I would have imagined. I took business classes and joined a business networking and mentorship group called Vistage to learn how to handle the finances, marketing, employees, insurance, overhead, inventory, and taxes. I spent months trying to find the right location, and then once I finally found it, another six months building it out. The learning curve was steep and fast.

Six months after my rejection from Baylor, I took a refresher course in sinus surgery at the University of Texas, Houston. One of the lecturers discussed a lab she was using to more accurately diagnose and treat patients with chronic sinusitis. The company, MicroGenDX, uses PCR (polymerase chain reaction) technology instead of the traditional method of culture to identify the bacteria living in the sinuses. I had never heard of this technique and was excited to use it. The standard of care at that time was to treat chronic sinusitis with a very strong antibiotic for four consecutive weeks (usually levofloxacin) without knowing which bacteria were causing the infection. When I started my new practice, I connected with the rep for MicroGenDX, Karl Mundt—Karl and MicroGenDX would play a pivotal role in my journey when COVID hit.

Money was not a motivating factor in returning to work. I approached the new venture with the goal of being a happy doctor with happy patients above all else. The cash-only model was untested and financially risky, but my intention was to break even and have high job satisfaction. I had extensive firsthand experience as a patient and knew how I could make going to the doctor a more patient-friendly experience.

The hardest part of starting my practice was finding the location. I ultimately ended up in a former dentist's office in a high-end strip mall close to the Texas Medical Center. Online critics have mocked me for my "strip mall" location, but I chose it very deliberately. Sick patients don't need the added stress of navigating a ten-story parking garage and two sets of elevators when trying to see their doctor. This served me very well during the pandemic when I was able to administer breathing treatments in people's cars.

I wanted the office to feel inviting and soothing, so I used spas for inspiration. We periodically infuse the air with peppermint spray and give patients a cold peppermint towel to clean their hands when they arrive. My waiting room plays spa music and is purposely very small. If there is a wait, patients are taken to a private area to relax in a zero-gravity massage chair. I don't have patients fill out any papers and don't allow my nurses to collect copious amounts of information that just gets repeated to me by the patient. I offer as much on-site diagnostics and treatment as possible to spare patients the inconvenience of scheduling services elsewhere. We do breathing treatments, allergy testing, sinus CT scans, and sleep testing. I have a phlebotomist for lab work and IVs, and when the pandemic hit, I offered rapid testing for COVID, flu, and other viruses.

I modified the existing dental equipment from the previous tenant to create a powerful sinus irrigation and suction device and trained my nurses on how to use it. Inspired by the experience in my in-laws' bathroom, I hired a massage therapist and trained her on using the sinus irrigation device. She created a relaxing and therapeutic sinus treatment with steam, irrigation, percussion, aromatherapy, and massage.

Though it had been in the making for over two years, I didn't get my practice open until six months before the pandemic started. At the time, my patient volume was low, and despite the slight uptick in bronchitis patients during spring break, I assumed my quiet clinic would stay that way. As a solo practitioner, I didn't have other doctors to talk to and didn't trust the media's version of events. I felt like an outsider, not part of the system, safe in my small, little, one-doctor clinic. I thought I would and could stay on the sidelines. In retrospect, I wish I had tried to learn everything I could have as soon as those first suspected patients came my way. After dipping my toe, I slowly waded into COVID, and eventually dove into it headfirst, but knowing what I know now, I waited too long.

CHAPTER 2

Early Lessons

It took 3,285 days—four years of medical school and five years of residency—for me to become a licensed, practicing otolaryngologist. The days were endless and mostly a blur, but the next to the last day—day 3, 284—twenty-four hours before I was released into the real world, I received advice that at the time seemed quite inconsequential. It would take twenty years to manifest, but day 3,284 changed the course of my life.

When I graduated in 2003 from residency at Stanford, I could never have imagined the events that have unfolded over the past five years. Work following graduation was considerably easier than my training, and when I joined the small private practice with two other ENTs in Houston, I anticipated a smooth, gentle career. Little did I know the seeds of chaos had already been planted.

Impactful experiences are often difficult, and at one point, I considered residency the hardest five years of my life. I learned not only what to do, but what not to do. I figured out whom to emulate and whom to disregard. I was pushed to my limits and considered quitting many times. Getting to the finish line seemed miraculous, and the day before graduating, apart from a few loose ends, I thought I had finally finished what felt like the longest marathon of my life.

That sense of closure was premature. Though it started like all others, the last day of my training turned out to be the most consequential day of my career. My team—myself as chief resident with four junior residents and a medical student—met early (5:30 a.m.) to round on patients on the floor and the ICU (intensive care unit). Physicians "make rounds" on patients in the hospital twice a day, collecting information from the nurses on their condition, talking to the patient, doing a physical exam, evaluating labs and imaging studies, and creating a treatment plan. As a team, we rounded morning and evening, and the attending (our teacher) typically only joined for evening rounds. Morning visits with patients were rushed, as we needed to be in the operating room by 7:15 a.m. Patients are not usually full participants in the day's plan, as time doesn't allow for much discussion. After rounds, I called my attending to update him or her on our patients while my team scurried to different operating rooms. As chief resident, I chose whom to operate with and on whom. Toward the end of my training, "with" became more important than "on whom"—each attending had a reputation, and I had my preferences.

With the advantage of rank, on this day I chose to do a parotidectomy (removal of the parotid gland, one of the glands located in the cheeks that secretes saliva) with Dr. Fee, the former head of the Department of Otolaryngology at Stanford University Medical Center. When he stepped down as department head, his position was filled by Dr. Goode, whom I mentioned earlier. They were oil and water; the two coexisted, and though I never saw outright conflict, I never sensed friendship. The dichotomy was educational. Dr. Fee was fast, decisive, and blunt. We all wanted to be in his operating room. Dr. Goode was innovative and exceedingly hard to please—the challenge to win him over motivated some of us. I never quite got there, but I appreciate him now. He died in October 2019; I really regret not knowing how he would have responded to the pandemic. He was exceedingly difficult to get along with. I suspect he would not have complied.

After surgery, we met for tumor board. Once a week, patients with head and neck cancer came to the clinic for evaluation by a full treatment team—surgeons, medical oncologists, radiation oncologists, and pathologists. Following their visit, we convened around a large conference table, presented each patient's history, and debated the treatment plan. It was professional, inspiring, and memorable, and one of the things I miss most from my training.

Journal club met weekly, where we dissected peer reviewed scientific articles. Each study faced relentless scrutiny—low power, weak controls, lack of randomization—and was often deemed unworthy. I don't recall specific articles, but residency left me with a deep skepticism of published research. As residents, we were complicit in our attendings' rush to publish, a necessity for their academic advancement. Quality frequently suffered, though we observed this silently. I learned that all studies require clinical correlation, and I placed greater trust in my attendings' insights and my own clinical experience.

Interspersed throughout the day were consults—other medical or surgical services calling us to help with various ear, nose, and throat issues on patients in the emergency room or in the hospital—and were often in the middle of the night. They frequently resulted in emergency surgery, and the unpredictability of these requests were what made residency particularly exhausting.

Consults aside, the twilight hours were often the hardest. The engine roared to a stop, but the work was not done. After surgery, morning and evening rounds, tumor board, journal club, clinic, and consults, residents headed to their office to tie up loose ends. Despite the grandeur of the surrounding hospital, our little residents' office was smaller than most walk-in closets. The space was crammed with cubicles, dimly lit desks covered in paper charts, and x-ray jackets. This was 2003, and everything was pen and paper, no electronic charting or orders. We returned phone calls from patients and prepared for the next day, hunting down charts and films for the following day's surgery patients. Hunger and fatigue consumed us but had to be ignored, especially if staying overnight to take call.

Residency often felt like a prison sentence. Apart from the physical demands—sleep, food, and time off were luxuries—we felt mentally indentured. We were young and learning, and lives were often at stake, so we needed to fall in line. But after nine years of constantly doing and saying as told (for my specialty of otolaryngology, it was four years of medical school and five years of residency), most of us felt defeated and ready to get out. That year, all three of us graduating chief residents chose to go into private practice rather than extend our training with a fellowship or work in academic medicine—a sign that we had all had enough.

Entering private practice after residency was often viewed as a step down. Academic physicians saw private practitioners as less competent, as they often refer complex cases to academic centers. As residents, we questioned their capabilities, rolling our eyes at transfers from private ENTs and judging the referring physicians. After transitioning to private practice, I realized the issue wasn't always the doctors but the systems they worked in. Complex head and neck cases require specialized equipment and trained nurses, often unavailable in private hospitals. I learned this quickly once I graduated—my very first night on call, I was summoned to the ER to see a two-year-old who had swallowed a coin. The coin was stuck in his esophagus, so I took him to the OR at a small private hospital in the middle of the night only to learn they didn't have the equipment I needed—a rigid esophagoscope. I improvised, removed the coin, and silently apologized to all the private ENTs I had judged during training.

The final days of residency are met with mixed emotions. Relief to have survived is at the forefront, but trepidation as to what lies ahead lurks in the background. Looking back, it takes a bit of courage to leave the safety of academic medicine, where an enormous team is always there ready to help. My education prior to this point was purely scientific. No one discussed life on the outside. I didn't know what I didn't know, probably because my attendings, never having left the hallowed and sheltered halls of academia, didn't know either.

I received the most valuable piece of practical advice one day prior to graduation—day 3,284 of 3,285 of my training—when Dr. Fee popped into the residents' room during those exhausting twilight hours. The room was our haven, and attendings rarely entered. He had our immediate attention.

His golden retriever, who came to work with him daily, accompanied him into the room. Dr. Fee got right to the point. "Guys, I want to wish you well and give you some advice. First, find out who the best doctors are in your area, and keep a list so you know whom to refer your patients to. Your patients will judge you based on the quality of doctors you send them to. Second, when new medications come on the market, don't rush to use them. Give them time. Wait to see if there's a fallout before prescribing them."

There may have been more, but if so, I don't remember. For some reason, this last piece of advice stuck with me and—twenty years later—changed my life in ways I never would have imagined.

CHAPTER 3

Early Mistakes

My medical training never included discussions about the FDA (Food and Drug Administration). I knew they regulated prescription drugs, but until the pandemic, never gave the agency any thought. Dr. Fee's admonition to proceed with caution before prescribing newly approved medications seemed wise, but it didn't cause me to question the integrity of the FDA. I never imagined this government agency would become relevant in my practice.

My first exposure to Big Pharma corruption came shortly after leaving Stanford, when I learned one of my prior attendings nearly died after taking Vioxx. He was suffering from lower back pain, and when the pain intensified, he was misdiagnosed with cancer. After major exploratory surgery, he was found to have severe bleeding around his kidneys consequent to taking Vioxx. After five years, Merck withdrew Vioxx from the market because of concerns about cardiovascular risks, and a meta-analysis published in *The Lancet* concluded the drug should have been pulled off the market several years earlier. Merck was fully aware of the problems and tried to cover them up.[1] I recently met a former drug representative for Vioxx who attested to this.

I practice medicine far differently now than I did when I first got out of residency. As a young doctor, I was much more cavalier about starting patients on long courses of treatment, and despite Dr. Fee's advice, using brand-new drugs at the behest of drug reps who inundated us with samples. Using samples saved patients the cost and hassle of going to the pharmacy, and thanks to the one-sided information from the drug reps, I thought I was using the best medications available.

I was trained to treat patients with chronic sinusitis with four weeks of a very strong antibiotic—typically the fluoroquinolone levofloxacin—but in the early years of post-residency practice, I often used their upgraded version, Avelox. Fluoroquinolones have been on the market for fifty-plus years, but the FDA did not publish safety concerns until 2008, when it issued a black-box warning over increased risk of tendonitis and tendon rupture.[2] In 2013, the FDA changed the labeling of fluoroquinolones to include an additional safety concern of permanent peripheral nerve damage,[3] and in 2016, issued the following statement, "We have determined that fluoroquinolones should be reserved for use in patients who have no other treatment options for acute bacterial sinusitis, (ABS), acute bacterial exacerbation of chronic bronchitis (ABECB), and uncomplicated urinary tract infections (UTI) because the risk of these serious side effects generally outweighs the benefits in these patients."[4] Two years later, in 2018, the FDA sent out an additional warning of increased risk of aortic rupture[5] in certain patients.

Trovafloxacin was a popular new fluoroquinolone approved by the FDA in December 1997, but it was withdrawn from the market in May 2000 after 140 cases of severe liver "events" and fourteen cases of acute liver failure. I was in residency at the time and remember prescribing it. Thankfully none of my patients suffered liver failure, but over time, I realized the side effects of these antibiotics could be quite severe and became much more cautious about prescribing them. Now I rarely use them and am a bit horrified at how often I prescribed them in the past.

Another regrettable prescribing habit I developed during residency was putting patients on indefinite courses of proton-pump inhibitors (PPI's) for "silent reflux." Patients will often see an ENT for tightness in their throats, a symptom we call "globus." When their exam shows swelling in the larynx with no other explanation for their symptoms, most ENTs will empirically put patients on strong stomach acid blockers with the presumption that acid is refluxing from their stomach to their larynx and causing constant inflammation. Many of these patients don't have symptoms of heartburn, gas, or stomach pain, but the treatment completely shuts down their acid production nonetheless. Patients being treated for globus pharyngitis are placed on these medications, often at twice the recommended dosage, for indefinite periods of time. I remember reaching out to Dr. Fee when I was out in private practice, questioning this treatment strategy. Everyone was doing it, and though I don't recall his exact response, I believe he didn't see a problem with it. Since I started my new practice, I am much more conservative and can't recall a single patient I've recommended take PPIs. If stomach acid and reflux are a concern, I start with diet changes, elevating the head of bed, and Tums. In line with my instincts, a study published in 2021 from the journal *Cureus* stated, "widespread PPI use has led to emerging evidence of long-term adverse effects not described previously, including increased risk of kidney, liver, and cardiovascular disease, dementia, enteroendocrine tumors of the gastrointestinal tract, susceptibility to respiratory and gastrointestinal infections, and impaired absorption of nutrients."[6]

The pandemic was the first time I bothered to question the FDA and their drug approval process, and what I discovered was alarming. The majority of pivotal trials forming the basis for FDA approval enroll fewer than one thousand patients with a follow-up of six months or less, and post-market safety events are quite common amongst FDA-approved drugs. In the last four years, I've seen a large number of patients who suffered sudden onset of new medical problems shortly after receiving the COVID shot. I've never seen complications like this from any other pharmaceutical product on the market, probably because historically, the FDA has removed products in a timely fashion when problems arise.

A study published in the *Journal of the American Medical Association (JAMA)* in 2017 showed one-third of the 222 medications approved by the FDA between 2001 and 2010 were flagged for safety concerns, and it took a median of 4.2 years for these safety concerns to come to light.[7] Of these 222 approved drugs, sixty-one incremental boxed warnings were placed on forty-three, and three products were removed from the market entirely.

Another study looking at 548 products approved from 1975 to 1999 showed "56 (10.2%) acquired a new 'black box' warning or were withdrawn from the market. Forty-five drugs (8.2%) acquired 1 or more black box warnings and 16 (2.9%) were withdrawn from the market." The authors estimated that the probability of a new drug "acquiring a new black box warning or being withdrawn from the market over [a period of] 25 years was 20%." Further, half of eighty-one changes to drug labeling occurred within seven years of drug introduction to the market, and half of the drug withdrawals occurred within two years.[8]

Thanks to the National Childhood Vaccine Injury Act of 1986, vaccines are immune to all liability, making them a protected class of drugs with no legal guardrails. The FDA is solely responsible for oversight, and though they did their job in the past, none have been scrutinized or withdrawn since 1999. Looking at their history, vaccines, like all pharmaceutical products, have had safety issues, with some notable mishaps in oversight requiring removal from the market.

In 1955, a batch of polio vaccines from Cutter Laboratories infected 250 people with the virus and caused paralysis in many.[9] Despite the recall, years later another issue arose. Between 1955 and 1963, polio vaccines were found to have been contaminated with SV40 (simian virus 40). SV40 is a naturally occurring virus that infects monkeys, and rhesus monkey kidney cell cultures were used for the production of the vaccines. SV40 is considered an oncogenic virus, meaning it can induce tumors in some hosts and has been linked to certain types of human cancers, including brain tumors, bone cancers, malignant mesothelioma, and non-Hodgkin's lymphoma.[10] Between 10 percent and 30 percent of polio vaccine batches produced and distributed between 1955 and 1963 were contaminated with SV40.[11] The discovery of SV40's oncogenic nature in hamsters sparked concern about potential human health risks, leading to the recall of Salk vaccine in 1961 and the eventual discontinuation of Sabin's oral vaccine in 2000. Recent evidence has shown the COVID shots contain SV40 and was cited by Florida Surgeon General, Dr. Joseph Ladapo, as one reason to stop administering the shots.[12]

In 1976, forty-five million people, or 25 percent of the US population, received the swine flu vaccine, but after thirty-two Americans died and hundreds contracted Guillain-Barré syndrome, it was swiftly pulled off the market.[13] Months after inception, the swine flu immunization program was officially halted on December 16, 1976.[14]

In 1999, the first vaccine for rotavirus was removed following increased incidence of intussusception, a rare type of bowel obstruction, with the risk soaring to twenty to thirty times over expected risk within two weeks of receiving the vaccine. RotaShield vaccine was recalled in October 1999 after 101 confirmed and presumed cases of intussusception were reported to the Vaccine Adverse Event Reporting System (VAERS). Ultimately, "fifty-two patients required surgery, nine required bowel resection, and one patient died."[15]

This was the last action taken against a vaccine, but in the years since this occurred, the CDC pediatric vaccine schedule has exploded. Prior to 1986, children were routinely given DTP, (diphtheria, tetanus, pertussis), MMR (measles, mumps, rubella), HiB (Haemophilus influenza type B), and OPV (oral polio). Today, that list has expanded to include hepatitis A and B, varicella, PCV13 (pneumococcal conjugate), HPV (human papilloma virus), MCV4 (meningococcal conjugate), influenza, rotavirus, and COVID.

Apart from Dr. Fee's advice at the conclusion of my training, I was never educated to scrutinize the FDA, much less vaccines, and like many things I learned during medical school and residency, I assumed if the FDA approved a drug or a vaccine, it must be safe. It wasn't until the pandemic that that assumption was challenged.

CHAPTER 4

Dipping My Toes into the Pandemic

I know a few people who called things right from the very beginning of the pandemic, and I have the utmost respect for them. Alas, I wasn't as quick to catch on as I would have liked and have a few regrets over things I wish I had done differently. When the pandemic started, my clinic had only been open for six months, and I had a very quiet practice. As a solo practitioner who had been out raising kids for a while, I didn't have a network of physicians to communicate with. The events in the news seemed remote, and I did not anticipate that I would be seeing many COVID patients.

During the pandemic, common sense and an open mind proved to be a better guide than my elite Stanford education. We were facing a new disease with no standard of care, and prior to COVID, most physicians, including myself, believed viruses couldn't be treated. Before I knew about monoclonal antibodies, hydroxychloroquine, and ivermectin, I focused on treating the symptoms and covering for secondary bacterial infection, using breathing treatments, antibiotics, and steroids. I believe we all craved guidance on how to treat this novel infection. The majority of physicians unfortunately put their faith in government doctors with no clinical experience, strategizing from the safety of their homes over Zoom calls. I have always been independent-minded, and with the early success I was having in treating COVID patients, I grew more confident in going down a path different from what the FDA and CDC were calling for.

That being said, the seeds of skepticism planted during my early years of practice didn't sprout right away. Initially, I complied with mask mandates, even though I knew it made no sense to wear a mask while walking to a restaurant table only to remove it when seated. I still regret following that absurd rule. Early on, I was far too open-minded about the "vaccine," and in response to a mandate from Houston Methodist Hospital, almost got it myself. Thankfully, I never did.

When I returned to work in 2019 and started my own practice, I decided to approach treatment of chronic sinusitis differently from how I was trained. The standard of care was to put everyone with chronic sinusitis on four weeks of a broad-spectrum antibiotic, and if that failed, perform sinus surgery on them whether or not their CT scan showed anything structurally wrong. This approach never sat well with me, as it often failed, and it's very discouraging to operate on someone and have them tell you it didn't help.

PCR testing for chronic sinusitis was an important breakthrough allowing targeted antibiotic therapy. The alternative, sinus cultures, are notoriously inaccurate with low sensitivity; few ENTs use them. The PCR test is much more sensitive, with the caveat that it also picks up nonpathogenic bacteria that don't need to be treated. Our noses are not sterile, and not all bacteria are harmful. With experience, however, I became quite proficient in interpreting the results, and I have found it to be an invaluable resource in treating patients with chronic sinusitis. The same lab, MicroGenDX, developed a PCR saliva test for COVID and was the first lab I was aware of to offer COVID testing other than Labcorp.

Labcorp began offering a PCR COVID test via nasal swab on March 5, 2020, but most people weren't aware of this. The CDC led people to believe it was only available to certain people through the health department. Doing my own research, I discovered I could perform the test from my office and send samples to Labcorp, and we started using it on March 13, 2020. Four days later, on March 17, 2020, I sent the following email to Arian Campo-Flores at the *Wall Street Journal* regarding the availability of the test.

> I am an ENT in Houston and I think the public should know that Labcorp has had the test for COVID-19 since March 5th. Following the CDC, I assumed the test was only available to certain people and those people had to get tested through the health department. It was only through doing my own research that I figured out Labcorp had the test and have been testing people in my office since Friday.
>
> Thanks,
> Mary Bowden

He didn't respond.

Because they were the only lab in the country with the test, Labcorp soon became overwhelmed. Initially we received results back in one to two days, but as cases surged, turnaround time increased to two weeks. Meanwhile, the health department covering the largest medical center in the world, Harris County Public Health, could not keep up with demand. Even as late as six weeks after the pandemic, they were forced to ration testing. On April 29, 2020, they limited testing to those in close contact with someone diagnosed with COVID, those who had other health conditions (diabetes, lung disease, heart disease, pregnancy), those sixty and older, or those who were residents of nursing homes. Testing of asymptomatic patients was only allowed if they believed they had been exposed to COVID and were either part of an investigation of a cluster or an outbreak or were healthcare workers/first responders.

My clinic quickly ran out of swabs and couldn't get more, so we used an alternative test method, approved by Labcorp, of irrigating the nose with saline and having patients blow their nose into a cup. Because my clinic was one of the few in the area offering testing, demand was extremely high. The entire interventional radiology department (and their spouses) from the VA hospital showed up for testing one afternoon. Labcorp was taking two weeks to return results, and following this rush of testing, I had multiple angry and panicked doctors pounding on our doors after hours demanding their results.

I was fortunate to find an alternative to Labcorp, and on March 24, 2020, we implemented MicroGenDX's PCR saliva test as another option to Labcorp's test. It eliminated the need for swabs, which were difficult to find when demand exploded for testing. It also allowed us to test without coming in close contact with patients, and patients much preferred it due to the noninvasive nature. My clinic—located in a strip mall—was well-situated to test people in this manner. We handed the patient a sterile cup, labeled with their information, which they took to their car and spit into until the saliva reached a line. When finished, they left the cup in a basket outside the clinic door with a sign informing them of when they could expect results. At the end of the day, we FedExed all the specimens to the lab, and results typically came in the following evening. I personally texted every patient with those results. MicroGenDX did not accept insurance and charged us for each test; we charged the patients and provided receipts the patients could submit to their insurance company for reimbursement.

The local news ran a story on us, as initially we were the only place in town providing testing with such fast turnaround. As the news was keen to point out, our tests were not free, but the free tests were taking two weeks to get results. With the expectation to quarantine until results returned, these free tests were essentially worthless since everyone getting the test had to quarantine for fourteen days anyway.

I started tracking my percent positives and posted the results on Facebook and Instagram—I didn't become active on Twitter until much later. I was a member of two private groups on Facebook—West University Information Trading and Houston Women's Physicians Group. I'm relying mostly on memory because I was eventually kicked out of both groups, as well as Instagram, but at that time, I was posting weekly graphs of my percent positives on these forums.

My results mirrored closely what the health department was seeing, but I was quickly accused of fearmongering (if the percent positives were high) or downplaying the severity (if the percent positives were low). I made very little commentary, just posted the graphs, but people were outraged. I was called a grifter because I charged for the tests and used an "unapproved" method for testing. The government experts were the sole authority from the start; as a mere community doctor, my findings were automatically discredited.

With time, and as demand increased, I couldn't call everyone who was positive, and I discovered ways to streamline the process using a program called SimpleTexting. This helped, and I enjoyed the process of learning how to make the system more efficient, but doing it night after night, especially with four young boys at home, was stressful. Delays invariably occurred, usually from FedEx not being able to deliver the specimens to the lab on time, but occasionally from the lab or errors on our part, and some patients would get very upset. Most of the panic came from travelers who couldn't depart on a trip without the results. Those situations were memorable but thankfully rare.

I adjusted the price of the test according to what the lab was charging us but kept it between $150–200. We expanded to offer antibody and T cell blood testing when those became available, and in May 2020, I went to a nearby urgent care center to get a test we didn't offer—a rapid finger stick antibody test. The process took about twenty minutes, I never left my car, and I answered a series of questions from a nonphysician dressed in a hazmat suit. I told the person running the test that I was a physician and didn't have insurance, and she kindly told me not to worry about paying.

A week later, I received a bill from the facility for $2,720. The facility charged me as if I had seen an ER doctor.

STATEMENT OF ACCOUNT

Guar. Acct Nbr:

Description	Charges	Credits	Balance
Provider: JOHNSON NIA			
020 Discharge Date: 04/28/2020			
ER VISIT LEVEL 2 W/PROCEDURE	2,720.00		
Sub Totals:	$2,720.00	$0.00	$2,720.00
Grand Totals:	$2,720.00	$0.00	$2,720.00
Account Credit:			
PATIENT BALANCE DUE:			**$2,720.0**

Shocked, I posted it on my neighborhood Facebook site; the facility caught wind and told me I didn't need to pay. This kind of veiled upcharge for medical services is not unique to COVID, and it's one of the reasons I don't contract with insurance companies. Transparent, readily available pricing prevents fraud and profiteering. Later I reported this to the Texas Medical Board, but they chose not to investigate.

The more popular I became in the neighborhood, the more pushback I received; the members of Houston Women's Physicians Group on Facebook were particularly vicious. I realized I was a target and was worried they would make false reports to the health department to try to shut me down. I never made other people wear a mask, but I was careful about wearing one myself in the clinic for that reason. The governor of Texas, Greg Abbott, issued a mask mandate for health care workers on May 1, 2020:

All physicians providing patient care or engaging in an in-person patient encounter, must implement the following minimum COVID-19 standards of safe practice. (I) a mask must be worn by both the patient and physician or the physician's delegate when in proximity of the patient (meaning less than a 6-foot distance between the patient and the physician or the physician's delegate).[1]

My fears about being caught without a mask were not unfounded. An ENT in Palestine, TX, Dr. Eric Hensen, was reported to the Texas Medical Board for not wearing a mask in his clinic. He subsequently lost his license—eventually it was reinstated but only after a lot of unnecessary expense and stress.

In the early part of the pandemic, I was immersed in testing and extremely busy. Because we were the only place in town offering noninvasive testing with fast turnaround, demand was high, and I expanded our testing services to seven days a week. Every night I personally managed the communication of results, waiting by the computer to receive them from MicroGenDX, then sending out text messages to the patients. Initially, I called people who tested positive. It felt very serious and not the sort of thing that should be casually relayed by a text message. I hated those early calls because I didn't know what to tell them to do, and for those who weren't already my patients, I advised them to contact their primary care providers.

My first case came in right before spring break. A friend of mine's teenage daughter had just returned from a school trip in China. She was otherwise healthy but had bronchitis that wouldn't quit. I asked her and her mother if they had heard of the virus coming from China, but we all dismissed it as the possible cause of her illness.

A handful of patients trickled in after spring break, having caught the virus at ski resorts. Not knowing what I was fully dealing with, I used common sense and treated the symptoms. The majority of patients complained of tightness in the chest, so I used steroid breathing treatments, and if that wasn't enough, I tried oral steroids and antibiotics. These patients all survived, though some of them were challenging and didn't respond as quickly as I would have expected. In July 2020, one of my patients told me about Dr. Richard Bartlett's success with budesonide breathing treatments, and it was reassuring to hear others were using the same common-sense approach. Dr. Bartlett is an emergency room physician in Odessa, Texas, who made a YouTube video about this "simple solution to a complex problem," calling it a "silver bullet." After the video went viral, YouTube removed it, and Dr. Bartlett was turned in to the Texas Medical Board. He received four complaints against him in response to his advocating budesonide breathing treatments; all were eventually dismissed, and years later, studies were published vindicating his approach.[2]

I saw doctors on Houston Women's Physicians Group complaining about breathing treatments spreading COVID, so out of an abundance of caution, I ordered portable, battery-operated nebulizers and primarily administered breathing treatments in people's cars. Sadly, emergency rooms and hospitals were denying these to COVID patients for fear of spreading the virus. I thought giving the treatments in people's cars would be well received by both patients and other doctors as a way to keep people out of the emergency rooms, but to my frustration, they never really caught on. I also had patients take the nebulizer machines home and not return them, so I eventually moved the treatments back inside my office. I started prescribing the machines to COVID patients and sold them in my office, as pharmacies often didn't have them in stock. To this day, I still tell high-risk patients to have a machine at their house because I'm certain many patients could have stayed out of the hospital if they'd been able to do breathing treatments at home.

On March 17, 2020, we tested sixteen people for COVID. A week later, we tested eighty. In between those dates, President Trump declared hydroxychloroquine a "game-changer,"[3] and Dr. Zev Zelenko became famous for the YouTube video he sent to President Trump regarding his protocol of hydroxychloroquine, azithromycin, and zinc.

I didn't know about ivermectin early on, but I personally used hydroxychloroquine with great success. Following the influx of doctors from the VA who came in for testing, I developed a cough and tightness in my chest. Despite testing negative for COVID, my symptoms responded very quickly to hydroxychloroquine.

The day we tested eighty patients, March 26, 2020, the Texas State Board of Pharmacy (TSBP) proclaimed it was limiting prescriptions of chloroquine, hydroxychloroquine, mefloquine, and azithromycin in response to reports that hospitals and prescribers were stocking up on some of those drugs "even though they are not proven to treat COVID-19 effectively."[4] This not only deterred me from treating patients with these drugs, but it also deterred me from treating patients in general. If patients asked me to help, I did... but I didn't offer unless asked.

Under the TSBP temporary rule, prescriptions for those drugs were allowed only if they came with "a written diagnosis from the prescriber consistent with the evidence for its use." [5] The rule also limited new prescriptions for those drugs to a fourteen-day supply and prohibited refills without a new prescription or medication order.

Prior to COVID, I had never had to give a diagnosis to a pharmacist as a contingency to have the prescription filled. I had rarely encountered difficulties getting prescriptions filled, though one incident in 1999 demonstrated the senseless authoritarianism often seen in medicine, particularly in academic centers. I was a first-year resident in otolaryngology at the University of Texas Medical Branch and had prescribed my boyfriend the now over-the-counter antihistamine Allegra. We pulled up together in the drive-through to pick it up, and I suppose my youthful looks raised suspicions. After a series of questions, the pharmacist called my residency director (an administrator, not a physician), and even though I had a medical license, the residency director told the pharmacist not to fill it. The pharmacist complied.

The Texas State Board of Pharmacy restricted hydroxychloroquine use for outpatients but permitted it in hospitals. On March 28, 2020, the FDA granted an emergency use authorization (EUA) requested by BARDA (Biomedical Advanced Research and Development Authority) for chloroquine and hydroxychloroquine from the Strategic National Stockpile to treat hospitalized COVID patients when clinical trials were unavailable or participation was not feasible.[6] However, this EUA was short-lived, and the FDA revoked it on June 15, 2020.[7]

Hospitals stopped treating COVID patients with it; prescribing rights volleyed back to the outpatient doctors, as the TSBP rule expired on July 17, 2020. The establishment would not stand for that, though, and with lightning speed, Texas Medical Association's COVID-19 "Task Force"[8] swept in to issue an unenforceable, yet consequential, declaration recommending against the use of hydroxychloroquine for prevention or treatment of COVID. Though they had no regulatory authority, as the largest medical association in the country, their word was taken as standard of care.

Drs. Stella Immanuel, Richard Urso, Simone Gold, and others from America's Frontline Doctors protested in front of the Supreme Court on July 29, 2020. The video of Dr. Immanuel's speech touting the efficacy of hydroxychloroquine was retweeted by President Trump. After going viral, it was flagged as "misinformation" and taken down. I didn't see this video or know about it until much later. Five years later, I was honored to be invited to speak with the same group back on the steps of the Supreme Court in memory of that historic day.

Despite all the testing I was doing, most people were not seeking me out for treatment early on. Due to all the commotion surrounding hydroxychloroquine and azithromycin, I wasn't confident I could successfully treat them anyway and didn't offer unless asked. I mistakenly assumed their primary care doctors would help them. But with time, I noticed a worrisome trend as more and more people told me their doctors had either closed their office completely or said there was nothing they could do and to just go to the emergency room if they couldn't breathe. As crazy as it now sounds, the statement, "I tested positive for COVID so my doctor can't see me," became quite common.

Like firefighters running from a fire, many primary care doctors abandoned their patients in their time of greatest need. Doctors assume the risk of contracting infections from their patients when they earn their degrees; there is no clause stipulating they may run from their patients for fear of getting sick. My qualifications for treating COVID patients have been endlessly questioned, the critics claiming as an ENT, COVID is outside my area of expertise. On the contrary, I would argue that as experts in upper respiratory tract infections, *all* ENTs should have tried to treat COVID patients. And though I was quite comfortable doing so, I never would have needed to treat COVID patients if primary care doctors had done their jobs.

Until monoclonal antibodies became available, I relied primarily on antibiotics and breathing treatments. Demand for therapeutics was low, and we were so busy with testing that I didn't research alternatives to hydroxychloroquine as I should have. After hydroxychloroquine was essentially banned, ivermectin started to surface as an option, originally in Australia when Professor Thomas Borody reported success using it to treat twenty-four COVID patients. My brother-in-law, Army Perry, whose sister lives in Perth, sent me an email on August 21, 2020, about Borody's discovery. Unfortunately, I glossed over it. I don't know why, but I believe it was because I was so busy with testing and assumed, if it were legitimate, I would have heard about it from other physicians. I had no local doctors to collaborate with but was part of an online forum hosted by the American Academy of Otolaryngology. There was chatter on there about COVID but nothing about ivermectin. I looked through all my emails between March and December 2020, and the only email about ivermectin was from my brother-in-law Army! As Army astutely noted, "Best news of all, Bad Orange Man and Fauci have made no comments so it can't go political. Only be stopped by Big Pharma since it's also the fastest & cheapest solution available (about $2 a pill)." Ivermectin stayed under the radar far longer than hydroxychloroquine, but its days of infamy were certainly coming.

On November 16, 2020, the first monoclonal antibodies, Bamlanivimab from Eli Lilly, were distributed to hospitals but did not become available to doctors outside hospitals for three more months. Starting February 5, 2021, we enrolled a few patients in a study sponsored by Regeneron looking at the efficacy of their monoclonal antibody, and on February 27, 2021, I treated my first COVID patient with their product, REGEN-COV (casirivimab with imdevimab). We ordered the medication directly from AmerisourceBergen. The cost was absorbed by the government, we could order as many doses as we wanted, and they arrived within forty-eight hours. Medicare allowed physicians to charge a fee to cover the costs of administering the medication—supplies and staff—and reimbursed $310 per patient. We charged $175 and provided our patients with a receipt to get reimbursed by their insurance companies. Hospitals were making even more, as they charged a facility fee on top of the supplies and staff fee. I tried to find out how much Houston Methodist Hospital charged a cash-only patient for monoclonal antibodies, but despite multiple phone calls from myself and my staff, I never could obtain that information.

Monoclonal antibodies worked very well. Many patients felt worse the evening after treatment but woke up feeling tremendously better. I conducted surveys to gather data on outcomes. I recall one patient having to go to the emergency room for a possible seizure hours after his infusion, but otherwise, I did not see serious side effects. Ninety-eight percent of the patients who took my survey said they would recommend the treatment for a loved one.

Demand increased as word quickly spread of how well monoclonal antibodies worked, and Governor Ron DeSantis in Florida knew they worked too. During the COVID Delta variant wave, he set up easily accessible monoclonal antibody stations around the state, giving access to treatment for over one hundred thousand COVID patients. The federal government took notice, and in September 2021, the US Department of Health and Human Services (HHS) announced a dramatic reduction in the number of monoclonal antibodies to be allocated to states. DeSantis fought back, writing a letter to HHS Secretary Xavier Becerra and independently purchasing Sotrovimab from GlaxoSmithKline. Frustrated that Governor Greg Abbott in Texas was not doing the same, friends of mine urged me to do what DeSantis was doing—buy large quantities of monoclonal antibodies directly from the drug companies and stockpile them—but at $2,100 a dose, the cost was too prohibitive.

When the federal government reduced the supply of monoclonal antibodies to the states, the Texas Department of State Health took over distribution to physicians and hospitals in Texas. I didn't notice problems with supply until a few months later. On December 20, 2021, I received a surprising email from the health department: "I wanted to just let you know that your facility will be getting an allocation of 24 Regeneron and 36 of Sotrovimab shipped either this week or next week. I do not have a definitive date, however you should still receive the confirmation emails from ABC in regards to the shipping." That was the beginning of the end. Searching through old text messages, the most common text I sent my staff over the next few months was, "Do we have any monoclonal antibodies left?" Doctors were allowed to transfer monoclonals to other facilities in need, so I asked my nurses to call the hospitals. Around this time, we received a request from Houston Methodist to administer monoclonal antibodies to one of their VIP patients who didn't want to get treated in a hospital environment. We agreed on the condition that they share some of their monoclonal antibodies with us—they refused.

The government not only squeezed the supply but also called for restrictions on who could get treated. On December 27, 2021, New York implemented patient risk factors, including race and age, as criteria for treatment. Other states and many local facilities followed suit. Even though my supply was dwindling, I refused to do this, and only limited treatment to patients twelve and older since monoclonal antibodies were not approved for younger children. My clinic became known as a place to access monoclonal antibodies when other places refused.

During the winter of 2021–2022, the government stated monoclonal antibodies were no longer effective for the latest variant of COVID. On January 2, 2022, I sent a survey out to my patients and reported the results on January 6, sending out the following email to my patients:

The following data was collected from 60 people who received IV monoclonal antibodies for treatment of COVID within the last 3 weeks. All of them received Regen-COV.

Vaccination Status: 42% fully vaccinated, 52% not vaccinated, 5% partially vaccinated, 1% no response

Comorbidities: 10% with 3, 15% with 2, 25% with 1, 48% with none

- Severity of Symptoms: 7% severe... on the verge of going to the ER, 49% moderate... felt horrible but able to eat and drink, 44% mild... felt like they had a cold
- Other Medications: 40% Ivermectin, 6.7% Hydroxychloroquine, 93% Vitamin D, 95% Zinc, 93% Vitamin C, 43% Quercetin, 32% Inhaled Steroids, 22% Azithromycin, 33% Melatonin, 47% Aspirin

Response to Treatment: No patients required an ER visit or hospitalization. The 4 patients with severe symptoms all improved in 24–48 hours. 80% of the patients with moderate symptoms improved in 24–48 hours. The rest eventually recovered.

Conclusions: Based on this data, it is **premature to declare monoclonal antibodies ineffective against the Omicron variant**. We will continue to monitor and keep you updated. Unfortunately we are out of monoclonal antibodies again and do not know when we will get more.

With perfect timing, on January 21, 2022, the FDA expanded the use of Remdesivir to include nonhospitalized adults and pediatric patients (twelve years and older, weighing at least forty kg) with mild-to-moderate COVID. A day later, the Biden administration revoked the EUA for the original monoclonal antibodies, REGEN-COV and bamlanivimab/etesevimab, and pushed for states to pivot to other treatments—Paxlovid, molnupiravir, Sotrovimab, and

Remdesivir. One additional monoclonal antibody, bebtelovimab, did become available for nine months, starting February 11, 2022, but doses were exceedingly difficult to get. We received about five doses every one to two weeks, and by that time, I was relying primarily on ivermectin.

The FDA revoked EUAs for all monoclonal antibodies in 2022, but the EUA for the COVID shot remained active for almost 30 months following the official end of the COVID emergency (May 11, 2023).[9]

CHAPTER 5

Seeds of Controversy

I was nervous about using ivermectin. As stated earlier, I wish I had done my research sooner, but I was very comfortable with monoclonal antibodies, and they weren't controversial. When the government took over distribution and squeezed supplies, I was compelled to look to alternatives and remembered my brother-in-law's email. I had long ago decided not to use hydroxychloroquine since the pharmacists had issued an official restriction. The actual restriction did not last that long, but of course, many people, including myself, did not know that.

I started regularly prescribing ivermectin for COVID patients in the summer of 2021, nine months after the rollout of the shots, during the Omicron surge—the third surge to hit during the pandemic. In light of all the bad press on ivermectin, I decided to dig into its safety data and started with the FDA's website. Every prescription medication is indexed on their site, with the original studies submitted to the FDA at the time the drug was approved. Included in their database is toxicity information for each medication. I was particularly interested in finding the LD50 of ivermectin. The LD50 or "lethal dose 50" is a benchmark number used to define how toxic a medication is. In literal terms, it indicates the amount of drug needed to kill 50 percent of a particular lab animal. The lower the number, the more toxic the medication. The dosages we used to treat COVID are higher than those used to treat parasites, so I wanted to make sure these higher doses were safe.

The toxicity data is a bit buried but still accessible to the general public, and the LD50 ranges from 2.3 mg/kg in infant rats to 11.6 mg/kg in adult male mice up to 87.2 mg/kg in adult female mice. The doses we use for COVID patients are far below that, at 0.4 mg/kg.[1]

I took it one step further and performed a literature search on the NIH's database of peer-reviewed publications looking for studies on accidental or intentional overdoses with ivermectin. Consistent with the LD50 data, I was not able to find a single study, and at that point, was convinced ivermectin was extremely safe, even at the higher doses we were using for COVID.

I don't remember the first time a pharmacist rejected my ivermectin prescription, but the earliest text message I can find from a patient having trouble was August 16, 2021. "Long drawn out conversation with HEB pharmacist not wanting to dispense the ivermectin. Lee is sick. Finally have the ivermectin. Will keep you updated on his condition." Astounded, I sent this to a pharmacist friend and asked if pharmacists are allowed to not fill prescriptions. I had never encountered this before. "They have a right to, yes. Some are a-holes about it and it's a power trip. With ivermectin and hcq some are scared of losing their license," my friend replied.

As the controversy over ivermectin grew, the Texas Medical Board and the Texas State Board of Pharmacy issued a joint statement regarding prescribed drugs or treatment for COVID (September 3, 2021):

> The Texas Medical Board (TMB) and Texas State Board of Pharmacy (TSBP) do not endorse or prohibit any particular prescribed drugs or treatment for COVID-19 that meet the standard of care. Drugs are permitted to be prescribed off-label. It is the professional judgement of each physician to write their prescriptions while meeting all applicable federal and state statutes and rules. Similarly, each pharmacist must use their professional judgement in dispensing valid prescriptions while meeting all applicable federal and state statutes and rules.[2]

Nevertheless, every time I tried to send an ivermectin prescription to a big box pharmacy like Walgreens, HEB, Walmart, Kroger, or CVS, the pharmacist refused to fill it.

House Bill 2561, the Texas Pharmacy Act, passed in 2017, gave state pharmacists "exclusive authority" to determine whether or not to dispense a drug without having to explain why. Part of the original intent of the bill was to make it easier for pharmacists to refuse to serve patients who might be abusing painkillers. But language added allowed them to refuse to fill prescriptions on moral grounds. Sen. Van Taylor of Plano added exclusive authority, which gives pharmacists the final say.[3]

This bill had unforeseen yet dire consequences during COVID. Pharmacists with an agenda abused the spirit of the Texas Pharmacy Act to deny patients access to ivermectin. I found independent pharmacies who were happy to fill—"compounding pharmacies"—but most of them have limited weekend hours and don't accept insurance. A pill that costs pennies in Africa suddenly cost hundreds of dollars for a five-day course of treatment. I purchased my own ivermectin to give to patients who couldn't get timely access to a pharmacy, but even at wholesale, I paid four dollars for a 3 mg tablet.

Pharmacists are supposed to reach out to the physician if they have a concern about a prescription, but I have never had a single one contact me after rejecting my ivermectin prescription. When time allowed, I would call them to question why they wouldn't fill it. This was typically a fifteen-minute exercise, at a minimum, due to the long hold times and waiting for whoever answered to transfer me to the pharmacist. The most common excuse by far was, "The drug is not FDA-approved for COVID, and we aren't allowed to dispense it." I reported numerous pharmacists to the TSBP for refusing to fill my prescriptions, but none of them were investigated—they are protected by the Texas Pharmacy Act.

Prior to COVID, I rarely thought about the FDA. I knew they approved and regulated prescription drugs, but I was never trained to only use drugs according to their FDA-approved indication. During the pandemic, I had to defend "off-label" prescribing for the first time in my career. Most of the antibiotics I prescribe are technically "off-label," but I had never considered that prior to having difficulties prescribing ivermectin.

The problems really began in the spring of 2021 when the federal government, stepping on the toes of every doctor in America, directed the country not to take ivermectin for COVID. The attack started on March 5, 2021, with a newly published page on the FDA's website stating, "Ivermectin should not be used for the treatment or prevention of COVID-19."[4] To the unknowing public, this was interpreted as fact, but legally, the FDA does not have the authority to weigh in on treatment of medical conditions. The FDA's role is to approve prescription medications, not to regulate their off-label use or prohibit physicians from prescribing them for conditions they deem appropriate. The webpage omitted that physicians are legally permitted to prescribe ivermectin for COVID or other conditions off-label, a common practice in medicine. Additionally, the FDA released an FAQ titled, "COVID-19 and Ivermectin Intended for Animals,"[5] which emphasized veterinary formulations. While human and animal medications often share active ingredients, the FDA's framing suggested ivermectin was primarily an animal drug, misleading the public about its established use in humans. Mainstream media took this suggestion and ran with it, branding ivermectin far and wide as "horse dewormer."

Four days after the FDA published their webpage on ivermectin, the Biden Administration pressured Amazon to censor "anti-vax" books. Records subpoenaed by Rep. Jim Jordan (R-Ohio) and the House Judiciary Select Subcommittee on the Weaponization of the Federal Government show that on March 2, 2021, Andrew Slavitt, a former White House senior advisor for the COVID response, wrote to Amazon asking, "Who can we talk to about the high levels of propaganda and misinformation and disinformation of [sic] Amazon?" A week later, Amazon met with the White House, and immediately following this meeting, the company labeled "anti-vax books" as "Do Not Promote."[6]

The government's initial strike against ivermectin happened three months following the EUA approval for the Pfizer shot (December 11, 2020) as part of an orchestrated attack to combat "vaccine hesitancy." As of March 15, 2021, only 10 percent of Americans were considered "fully vaccinated." The overwhelming majority of Americans were reluctant to inject themselves with this novel product rushed to the market with no long-term safety data. Frustrated, Biden responded by announcing the deployment of a $1.5 billion PR campaign to combat "misinformation" and convince every American to get the shot. Ten days later, he upped the ante and announced an additional $10 billion would be poured into brainwashing Americans, particularly those in communities of color, rural areas, and low-income populations, to get the shots.[7]

Two weeks later, HHS officially announced the launch of this vaccine propaganda machine, calling it the "COVID-19 Community Corps." From their website:

> Today marks the launch of the national volunteer COVID-19 Community Corps, a U.S. Department of Health and Human Services (HHS) initiative to galvanize trusted messengers in the fight against COVID-19. Please help increase confidence in COVID-19 vaccines and encourage measures to slow the spread of the disease among your community by sharing your commitment to the COVID-19 Community Corps.[8]

Billions of dollars were doled out to influencers, community groups, and nonprofit organizations across the country. The list started at 275 recipients but grew to over 15,000, making the money trail virtually untraceable.[9]

At this point, 50 percent of Americans had had only one shot.

The same day the COVID-19 Community Corps was launched, April 1, 2021, a hospital in Texas made national news. Houston Methodist Hospital proudly declared it was setting a precedent—"leading medicine" as their tagline states—and mandating COVID shots for all of its employees. In June of 2021, the hospital fired 153 employees who refused to comply.

I had privileges at Houston Methodist but was not one of their employees—we had no financial relationship. Aside from the tour I took when I was granted privileges, I had never stepped foot in the hospital and only had privileges in case one of my patients needed to be hospitalized. Personally, I was extremely troubled by being told to get the COVID shots, but being so busy, I procrastinated on doing anything about it. At the time, I was not convinced it would work, but I still had enough trust in the government to not question its safety.

The hospital required everyone to sign an attestation that they were vaccinated or intended to get vaccinated by June 1, 2021, and when I signed it, I had every intention of getting the shot. I didn't make an appointment, but in the face of a looming deadline, woke up on a Saturday morning and just decided to get it over with. I searched online to find a nearby pharmacy with availability and ended up at a Kroger grocery store I had never been to before. The line at the pharmacy was long, and I grew impatient. I have a tendency towards impatience, and for once, it served me very well. I left, thinking I would go back another time—but with mounting firsthand evidence to fuel my doubts, I never returned.

I had many patients who worked at Methodist confide in me their reluctance to abide by their mandate. I sympathized and collaborated with other like-minded physicians to figure out how to help people get medical and religious exemptions. One easy stall tactic was monoclonal antibodies—the CDC advised the public to wait at least ninety days after receiving monoclonal antibodies to get the COVID shots.

COVID surged for the third time in the summer of 2021, nine months following the rollout of the shots, proving that the "vaccine" was not able to stop the spread of the virus. Because my clinic was doing a lot of testing, I saw the breakthrough cases and even reached out to Dr. Mas Takashima at Houston Methodist, asking him if he was seeing what I was seeing. My concerns were dismissed.

Mas is the chairman of the Department of Otolaryngology at Houston Methodist and a member of their board of directors and medical executive committee. Initially, he and I had a good relationship and were actually collaborating on research. In late March 2020, we formed a group to study ENT symptoms in patients with COVID. I provided the data from the patients I was testing and Mas's resident and medical student helped analyze it and write up the findings.

At the same time, I was working with MicroGenDX to compare the results of testing with a nasal swab versus their saliva test. On April 20, 2020, reporter Bill Barajas with local news station KPRC 2 ran a story about our study.

In emails to Mas and the group, I commented on what I was observing in these early patients we were testing. I saw patients testing positive long after symptoms had resolved and observed that none of the patients with classic COVID symptoms who tested negative ended up in the hospital, theorizing these patients were false negatives with less severe disease that was not clinically significant. I also noted that the test was not always necessary to diagnose—COVID is the only infection I've encountered that obliterates a person's sense of smell, but only temporarily. Prior to COVID, as an ENT I had often seen permanent loss of sense of smell after a viral infection, but this was the first time I saw a complete loss fully recover.

In mid-May, we submitted a request for IRB approval for our study, "Determination of Otolaryngologic Symptoms Among Patients with Laboratory-Confirmed COVID-19 in HMH Outpatient Setting." Despite the simplicity of the study, it took Houston Methodist's IRB over two months to approve it. IRB stands for "Institutional Review Board," and all researchers are required to submit their proposed studies through such an entity to make sure it meets ethical standards. Once it was finally approved, I had tested almost six thousand people and pushed to have all the data included, but I was met with resistance from Mas. I was particularly interested in studying the number of patients who tested positive but didn't have symptoms.

I wrote to the group, "Given how much data we have, I was thinking we'd look at data as a whole in terms of how outpatients present ... a couple of things that stand out that we could be looking at are the fact that family members rarely all test positive and that loss of taste and smell seems pathognomonic. I also have a huge number of asymptomatic patients, which is unique since most places have required symptoms to get tested." I also thought we should look at something no one else was looking at, remarking, "When I go to PubMed and search 'outpatient testing,' 'outpatient saliva testing' and 'families with COVID,' I don't get much. A search for 'anosmia (loss of smell) and COVID' brings up an abundance of articles." I was very curious why some members of a family didn't catch the disease from other sick members and was hoping my data would find an answer.

Mas responded, "With the wealth of data that you have, there is enough info for many separate papers! For this study, I think we should just stick with what we have and publish sooner rather than later as journals are still fast-tracking COVID articles. We can think of other studies and submit a different IRB for those."

As a retrospective case control study, we probably didn't need IRB approval, and it certainly didn't need to take two months to get it approved. I was sitting on mounds of data that could have led to some interesting conclusions, but instead, we were limiting our study to something so obvious that we really wouldn't be contributing anything to the understanding of COVID. As frustrated as I was, I was more compliant back then and didn't argue.

We initially submitted our paper to *The Laryngoscope,* and while waiting, we submitted an abstract, "COVID-19 Otolaryngologic Manifestations" to COSM (Combined Otolaryngology Spring Meetings), one of the annual academic meetings for otolaryngologists. An abstract is a brief summary of a paper, often presented on a large poster board at meetings prior to publication.

The findings were hardly groundbreaking and were obvious to everyone by the time we got IRB approval in July 2020. Of the 790 patients tested for COVID, eighty-eight tested positive. Nasal congestion (32.95 percent) and anosmia (28.4 percent) were the most common symptoms. Gustatory dysfunction (altered taste) was reported in nineteen patients (21.6 percent). Anosmia ($p<.01$), gustatory dysfunction ($p<.01$), fever ($p<.001$), and cough ($p=.042$) were significantly associated with COVID infection. The odds ratio of a positive COVID test among patients presenting with anosmia was 7.43.[10]

Even though I proposed the paper and gathered all the data, Mas asked to be senior author, citing this as a requirement on the part of the Houston Methodist IRB approval. We submitted the paper for publication to two different journals, but it was denied, probably because it took almost as long to get the paper written and submitted as the six months it took for the COVID shots to undergo testing and approval. Our findings were stale and uninteresting.

The summer after the COVID shots rolled out, I tried to publish a second study with Mas and another ENT on staff at Houston Methodist, Dr. Omar Ahmed, looking at changes in smell following vaccination ("Rapid Communication: The Risk of New or Recurrent Olfactory Dysfunction Following COVID-19 Vaccination"). This was a survey I sent out to over six thousand of my patients, but once again, I was excluded from taking the senior author position.

We were again paralyzed waiting for the Houston Methodist IRB committee to approve our survey. During that time, COVID was surging, and I sent two emails to Omar and Mas:

> I am seeing a huge uptick in positive cases but what is really surprising is that *the* majority of positive cases are in fully vaccinated people and the majority of these people have symptoms. Any buzz about this at Methodist or elsewhere that you have heard of?

I sent this on July 29, 2021, and when they didn't respond, I sent another email the following day: "Not sure if you've seen today's headlines about the high incidence of breakthrough cases in vaccinated people? The other interesting thing is that variant doesn't seem to be associated with loss of smell/taste. I have a feeling that by the time we get IRB approval, it will be old news!" Mas stayed quiet, but Omar did respond: "Very interesting, I think a majority of the patients hospitalized are unvaccinated. I guess the goal of the vaccine is to prevent against severe disease. I think it might be worthwhile studying these patients and evaluate for symptoms of smell loss in patients who were already vaccinated! Let me know what you think?—Omar"

I wanted to say a lot more but simply told him I would start tracking loss of smell in my vaccinated patients.

Omar wanted to send out another survey and emailed me on Sept 7, 2021:

> Hey Mary! We created a new survey with the intent of studying olfactory dysfunction in patients who *got* COVID-19 infection in the last 6 months who previously have been vaccinated and or received monoclonal antibodies. Here is the link to the new survey. Can you help get this out to as many patients as possible. How many patients do you think have tested positive for COVID-19 in the last 6 months at your clinic?
>
> *Thank you Mary! It has been so awesome working with you. —Omar*

I didn't hear anything about our three studies after this but followed up with Omar on November 29, 2021. He responded a few days later:

> Hey Mary, sorry for the delay, I was out of town. For one of the projects, there just wasn't enough number of patients to come up with any other substantial conclusions. One of the projects which we wrote up the paper, unfortunately it has gotten rejected 3 consecutive times.

I also emailed Mas, but he never responded. It's frustrating to look back at how much work I invested in those studies, how much data I had in my hands, and the missed opportunity to actually contribute to the understanding of COVID, but the experience was consistent with research projects I had worked on during residency. Academic centers are inefficient and slow to pivot. I knew we were wasting our time looking at anosmia in COVID patients but was powerless to do anything about it.

Mas stopped communicating about our research studies in July, but that would not be the last I would hear from him.

He never provided an adequate explanation of why I was seeing so many vaccinated patients testing positive, so I decided to start sharing my data on Twitter and Instagram.

I created a graph of our test results from the previous month of July, showing that sixteen people who were vaccinated tested positive and sixteen people who were unvaccinated tested positive. Of those, fifteen of the sixteen vaccinated patients had symptoms, whereas ten of the sixteen unvaccinated patients had symptoms. I had very few followers at the time, but I posted the graph in the comments of twenty-four accounts, some of which had a big following like Peter Hotez, Eric Topel, and the CDC. None of my posts received a single like.

At that point, I was not in the public eye. I posted test results on social media, and though I received some pushback from the neighborhood Facebook group West University Information Trading, I was mostly ignored.

In mid-August, I received a call from Karl Mundt, the rep for MicroGenDX (the lab we were

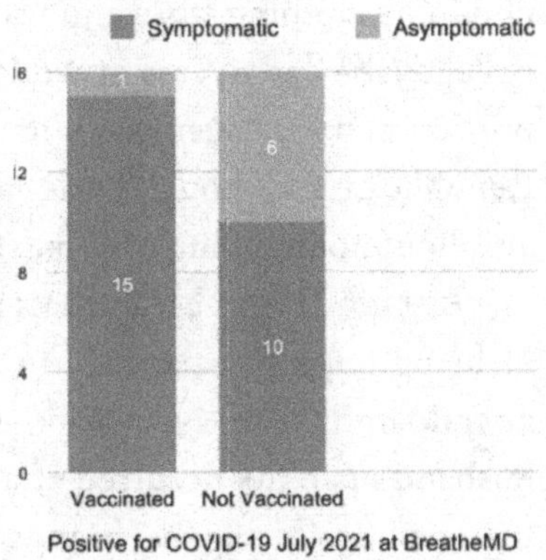

Positive for COVID-19 July 2021 at BreatheMD

using for our COVID testing), telling me Michael Berry wanted to interview me on his radio show.

"Who?" I asked.

"You don't know who Michael Berry is?" Karl asked in disbelief. Curious, I turned my car radio to the AM stations for the first time ever and caught his show. The intro exuded bold machismo, with the announcer declaring "locked and loaded" amid rolling drums and blaring trumpets. I was not surprised to hear a thick Texas accent when Michael started speaking.

In the decade prior to the pandemic, I considered myself politically agnostic. I voted for Trump but barely. I was quite fond of his reality TV show, but in my opinion, that made him seem a bit frivolous. I was so busy with my kids and working that I really didn't pay much attention to politics. I listened to NPR in the car on occasion and the rest of my news came from social media. I was, as Jesse Kelly described in an interview with Tucker Carlson, in "make-believe land" where I was completely disengaged from what was happening in the world around me. Medical school, residency, and raising four young boys were all-consuming, and I didn't make time to read anything outside of medicine.

Growing up, I never stopped working, starting with babysitting in middle school to working at my dad's hardware store and a local children's clothing store and waiting tables in high school through college. The early years of working hard and handing over a large portion of my meager wages to the government pushed me to vote Republican, and though I was hardly an activist, I felt fairly passionate about not handing over most of my paycheck to the IRS.

As I got older, I became less interested in politics, mostly because of being busy, but partially in response to marrying into a very liberal family from New York. My first introduction to my future husband's parents occurred at a dinner party with his parents and their politically aligned friends. At the time, I was a second-year resident and had very little flexibility in my schedule. I had an emergency come up just as I was due to leave for the party. My colleague took over, and I flew out of the ER to make it to their party on time.

I arrived late and a bit disheveled to a large table of well-heeled couples about thirty years my senior. The moment I sat down, my future mother-in-law fired her first shot. "Mary Talley, who do you plan on voting for in the upcoming election and why?" ("Mary Talley" is a double Southern name. My godmother's full name was Mary Talley, and her full name became my first and middle name. My oldest and closest friends call me "Mary Talley" rather than "Mary.")

At this point in my life, I've had hundreds of interviews, but only a few questions are seared in my memory—and my future mother-in-law's question is one of them.

Unprepared for the inquisition, my brain froze. I could barely remember who was running, and as all eyes bore down on me, I meekly uttered, "Bush." I didn't have an articulate reason why. I considered myself a Republican and didn't like the looks of Gore or his voice, but responding with that kind of levity wouldn't have worked in this crowd. I was surrounded by people who had very strong opinions, so I shut my mouth and slipped into the shadows of their efforts to outargue each other. In the ensuing engagement and marriage to their son, I'm not sure I ever emerged from that shell when the conversation turned to politics.

Twenty years later, when Michael Berry asked to interview me, I was still very reluctant to venture anywhere near politics. I strongly believed politics had no place in medicine, and I was concerned that, if I went on his show, my approach to treating COVID patients would be misconstrued as having political motivations. After weighing it over though, I decided a short discussion on what I was seeing and how I was treating patients could not possibly be viewed as political. At this time, I was not publicly known and not considered controversial.

When Michael called to introduce himself, I was on my back porch, separating myself from my children in the house, nervously pacing and careful to keep my volume low enough so the neighbors couldn't hear me. I had no idea what he looked like, but based on his voice, I envisioned a mix between Burt Reynolds and Al Pacino—charismatic, very Texas, and bold. I was wrong about his looks—he favors Billy Bob Thornton—but spot-on about his personality. I was quite reserved at the start of our call, but by the end of the conversation, I had stopped pacing and was sitting in my favorite Adirondack chair with my feet propped up on a side table.

He started by asking me basic questions, and as the conversation progressed, the questions became more personal. I remember a few details, but somehow, he correctly guessed the neighborhood I lived in. A large highway, known as the "loop," divides the city geographically and culturally, with the people living "outside the loop" voting more conservative than those "inside the loop." Not purposeful, but remarkably in line with what was happening in my life, I had recently migrated outside the loop—and Michael figured it out. I imagine I was a tough one to break—my walls are thick to begin with, and I had no experience with the media—but being a master at his profession, he earned my trust in that brief introductory conversation. Moments before our call ended, I asked him how long I'd be talking, and he said, "We'll see how it goes."

The interview fell on the day of my monthly Vistage meeting. I anticipated a ten-minute interview and decided to do it from my car in the parking garage of the meeting venue. I was nervous, particularly since I had never done a live interview, but figured I could get through ten minutes. At the time, I had no idea what a cult following Michael had.

The questions started off straightforward, and when the first commercial break came, he asked if I could stay for another segment. I hesitated because my meeting had already started but agreed. During the break he texted me, "Just relax. You're doing great. My audience loves you." I didn't believe him but smiled.

One thing led to another, and I ended up on the show for two and a half hours. My discomfort intensified with time, but during each break, he sent encouraging text messages. Toward the end, I remember feeling exhausted and wondering when it would be over. The questions got harder and less relevant to COVID, and I was nervous I was going to say something that would really get me in trouble. Michael can be very direct, which I appreciate, but I found it difficult to handle, particularly given my lack of experience with the media. At one point, he asked me if I had been in a sorority. Biting my tongue, I asked what that had to do with anything, and when the opportunity was right, I fired back by asking him if he'd ever had a pap smear. When it was over, I was convinced I had done a horrible job.

We are our own worst critics, and it took me a very long time to have the courage to listen to that interview. With the benefit of time, I now understand that he kept me on that long because the interview went well, at least in the minds of his listeners. He later told me, "I had sport going back and forth because you were obviously very smart and very accomplished, but very uncomfortable with me and that amused me." It felt like he was trying to break me on-air and scored points with his listeners when he succeeded. It was a tough way to get my feet wet, but like most challenges, it made me better. As the interview dragged on, I gradually forgot thousands of people were listening and started talking to him like we were having a private conversation. When he said things that were unexpected, I pushed back. Some said we sounded like an old married couple bickering.

Michael has invited me back several times since, but the dynamic has shifted. I'm more guarded now, like handling a loaded gun, careful to prevent it from going off unexpectedly.

I've done hundreds of interviews since, but his are by far the toughest. He wields humor unpredictably, tossing curveball questions that catch you off guard. You're left wondering whether to match his wit or stay steady and let him chuckle at his own jokes. Nevertheless, I look forward to the challenge when I get the opportunity and am certain I owe most of the support I've received in Houston to him and his listeners. When the city of Houston and the medical mafia came after me, Michael Berry was the first and loudest voice to stick up for me, and I'll be forever grateful for that.

CHAPTER 6

Hospital Prisoners

I got a small taste of publicity being on the Michael Berry show, receiving emails and calls of support from many Houstonians after the show. My practice picked up, and to this day, I regularly have patients come in because they heard that interview. At the same time, I noticed an uptick in animosity from the small private groups I belonged to on Facebook, West University Information Trading and Houston Women's Physicians Group. I wasn't even posting on Twitter at that point, but things were heating up on other social media platforms, and based on some of the comments directed toward me, I felt I needed to tread carefully.

In late summer 2021, 70 percent of Americans had received a COVID shot, yet COVID cases were surging for the third time since the pandemic started. The government's investment of over $11 billion in propaganda to combat vaccine hesitancy had not been as successful as hoped. That changed when the FDA posted a tweet on August 21, 2021.

The tweet featured two photos, a young, attractive healthcare worker nuzzling a horse alongside a photo of a doctor and patient facing each other, both wearing masks. The caption was unnecessary—the image conveyed the message loud and clear—but read, "You are not a horse. You are not a cow. Seriously, y'all stop it." In court, the FDA would claim this was merely a quip, but the "quip" set off a cascade of events with dire consequences. Those of us who treated COVID estimate as many as 85 percent of deaths attributed to COVID could have been avoided with early treatment, but thanks to the FDA's "quip," one of those treatment modalities became virtually inaccessible.

The tweet went viral, reaching twenty-four million eyes in the first week, and the media embraced it with gusto. Ivermectin became instantly branded as horse dewormer, not suitable for humans, and anyone who claimed otherwise—like famous podcaster Joe Rogan—was publicly attacked.

Two days later, on August 23, 2021, the FDA changed Pfizer's COVID shot, Comirnaty, from EUA to fully approved, a step required in order to initiate mandates. Comirnaty is not the version that was actually distributed, an important technicality that allowed Private First Class Derrick Wynne to fight back and win when he was dishonorably discharged from the Army for refusing the shots. After arguing the vaccine offered by the military was not the FDA-approved Comirnaty version, he successfully had his discharge upgraded to honorable, with benefits reinstated.

The day following the FDA's approval of the Pfizer shot, a flurry of big companies announced mandates for their employees, and the following day the Pentagon announced mandates for the military. In lockstep with the FDA, the CDC sent out a four-page health alert about ivermectin the same day the Pentagon announced its mandate.

The coup d'état occurred on September 9, 2021—nineteen days after the horse tweet—when Biden announced all businesses with one hundred or more employees must force their employees to get the COVID shots. The same day, physicians across the country received an email from the American Board of Internal Medicine, the American Board of Family Medicine, and the American Board of Pediatrics parroting a declaration made by the Federation of State Medical Boards (FSMB) that spreading misinformation could result in loss of license.

To tie up loose ends, HHS took over distribution of monoclonal antibodies on September 13, 2021. Whereas I once was able to get an unlimited supply, I was no longer able to get monoclonal antibodies to treat my patients.

The intention was clear. Shut down off-label prescribing of a safe, inexpensive, time-tested medication by branding ivermectin as only for horses. Threaten physicians who challenge the government narrative. Remove the most effective early treatment option available. No early treatment, plus no physician dissent, meant no choice but the COVID shot.

This did not deter me, but it certainly made my job harder. I never offered the COVID shots to my patients. Before I knew how dangerous they were, I entertained the possibility, but the storage requirements for COVID shots posed significant challenges, as they needed to be kept between -130°F and -76°F and could only remain at room temperature for up to two hours. This was an obstacle I could not see overcoming in my small office. I've often wondered about the stability of the vaccines administered at outdoor stadiums during the intense summer heat, where people lined up in their cars. When I asked Dr. Robert Malone about this, he suggested that heat exposure could cause the vaccine components to consolidate and thicken. The clinical implications of this are unclear, but he believed it could increase the potential for harm compared to vaccines stored at the required cold temperatures.

At this point, I had used ivermectin in over two hundred patients and was convinced it was both safe and effective. High-risk patients who took it early responded very well, and I was keeping those patients out of the hospital. The public was learning of the horrors going on in the hospitals, where people were treated like prisoners, given toxic medications without informed consent, and isolated from their loved ones. Patients who would have normally gone to the hospital but were terrified of what might happen if they did started showing up in my clinic.

Shortly after the FDA dropped its nuclear bomb on ivermectin, several very memorable patients entered my life and changed my understanding of COVID-induced respiratory disease. The most challenging patient was a sixty-two-year-old veteran with a history of severe coronary artery disease, having had two heart attacks as well as a prior history of throat cancer. He walked in, barely, with an oxygen saturation of 62 percent. I had excellent, like-minded nurses helping me at the time. One, Jennifer Bridges, was fired by Houston Methodist Hospital for refusing to get the COVID shots and led a large group of other employees in a lawsuit against them. Another, Kimberly Peeples, was fired by a highly reputable primary care clinic affiliated with Houston Methodist, the Sunset Clinic, also for not getting the shots. Jennifer and Kimberly knew the urgency of this patient's condition, quickly grabbed me, and we went to work.

Mr. Rodriguez had become ill seven days prior, and the course of his illness was familiar to me. The first week of symptoms was typical of a bad flu—sore throat, fever, headache, cough. Loss of smell and taste (anosmia) was pathognomonic, meaning the symptom was so unique that it alone was enough for diagnosis. People have argued that COVID was just the flu in disguise, but the flu doesn't cause this symptom. This was the first disease I had seen where the loss of smell was complete but not permanent. Other viruses can damage the olfactory nerve, but typically once this happens, the patient's sense of smell never returns. COVID was interesting in that it caused the sense of smell to completely vanish then miraculously return.

The eighth day of illness was typically the day people decompensated, and that was the day Mr. Rodriguez decided to come see me. He had tried to use the free medical care provided by the VA, but over the phone, they told him to just go to the emergency room if he couldn't breathe. That didn't sit well with him, and somehow, he found me.

I was encountering something I had never seen before in an outpatient clinic. Normally, if a person came in short of breath with an oxygen saturation below 90 percent, I would have called 911 and had an ambulance take the patient to the hospital. But Mr. Rodriguez was determined to stay out of the hospital. I believe in patient autonomy and honored Mr. Rodriguez's right to possibly die in my office.

We put him on oxygen, started an IV, and gave him a breathing treatment. I went to the Front Line COVID-19 Critical Care Alliance's (FLCCC) website and looked up their MATH+ protocol, a very detailed and well-researched list of medications and vitamins created by critical care doctors Dr. Pierre Kory and Dr. Paul Marik. Ivermectin was the mainstay, but a key addition was high-dose IV methylprednisone. Hospitals were using baby doses of a different steroid, dexamethasone, a medication that has been shown to be less effective than methylprednisone for respiratory distress. I threw the kitchen sink at him, adding high-dose vitamin C, B vitamins, zinc, glutathione, IV famotidine, ceftriaxone, oral ivermectin, melatonin, and aspirin, plus breathing treatments. He went home every night with oxygen and came back several days in a row for the same regiment of treatment. Miraculously, he survived. Two more patients like him followed soon after, and I realized these COVID patients were able to tolerate extreme levels of hypoxia that in other situations might have required intubation.

The FDA's smear campaign on ivermectin made it much harder for my patients to get a medication that is offered over the counter in other countries. I ordered my own to give to patients in a pinch, but Texas law prohibits physicians from dispensing more than three days of any prescription drug. With the help of patients, we created a list of pharmacies willing to dispense it, and soon we had a pharmacy from most areas of town. Patients started coming to see me before they got sick because they knew they might not be able to get the medications they needed in a timely fashion. I saw a significant number of families who wanted to have everything on hand in the event they came down with COVID. Never had I needed to do this in my career—help patients stock up on a medication in advance, not because it was in limited supply, but because their own government didn't want them to have it.

One family contacted me before traveling to Europe, requesting ivermectin to take with them in case they fell ill abroad. Their seventeen-year-old son, who had a history of kidney failure and a transplant, was a particular concern for them. Since ivermectin is metabolized by the liver and has no interactions with his medications, I agreed to prescribe it. Unbeknownst to me, I was communicating with the boy's father and stepmother. The boy's mother discovered the prescription and reported me to the Texas Medical Board, which pursued her complaint. After nearly two years and $16,105 in legal fees, the charges were dismissed. The child never even took the medication.

This experience was just one of many challenges I faced during the pandemic, a period that pushed me far beyond the stresses of my residency, which had been the most demanding time of my life until then. While my ENT career had been relatively calm after training, the pandemic brought unprecedented obstacles. Not only did I have to navigate treating a novel disease, but I also faced intense scrutiny and criticism from colleagues for my successful treatment approach, forcing me to defend it publicly. Though I had never been sued before, I quickly became acquainted with the legal system.

During my time as an ENT resident at Stanford, I published a study on informed consent.[1] Patients undergoing sinus surgery often believe it's simply a matter of cleaning out the inside of the nose, but because the sinuses are located in between the eyes and just under the brain, major complications, such as blindness, cerebrospinal fluid leaks, and meningitis are rare possibilities. Our study looked at whether or not it was necessary to disclose these risks to patients, with the hypothesis that because they are so frightening, patients might decide to forego surgery if they were aware of all potential risks.

I was not excited about this paper and only participated because I had to. I was trained that all potential complications, no matter how severe, had to be disclosed prior to surgery. I didn't see the need to subject it to statistical analysis and assumed we were just doing it to meet the attending's annual publication goals. No surprise, the patients overwhelmingly wanted to know all the risks. Looking back, I'm shocked this study didn't raise eyebrows internally; our attending seemed hopeful to prove hiding information from patients prior to surgery was permissible.

Like the tidbit of advice I received from Dr. Fee, this seemingly minor educational experience would take twenty years to bear significance. Though writing the paper didn't really teach me anything I didn't already know, it foreshadowed the brazen violations of human rights that occurred during the pandemic. I never imagined the issue of informed consent would bear such significance in modern times. Eighteen years after publishing the article on informed consent and sinus surgery, I published a similar article, this time based on actual rather than theoretical events surrounding the issue of informed consent.[2]

Medical ethics are part of every medical student's education—but not a key focus. I recall thinking the mistakes of our predecessors seemed blatantly obvious and not something I'd likely encounter again. That assumption was shattered during the pandemic, when people were forced to choose between taking an experimental gene therapy with no long-term safety data and keeping their jobs or staying in school. Two fundamental pillars of medical ethics, informed consent and patient autonomy, were completely disregarded during COVID. I am certain future generations will look back on this time in our history with disbelief and horror.

Respect for patient autonomy not only includes allowing patients to refuse medical interventions and treatments, but also to choose which interventions and treatments they receive. Patients must be given options. This is fundamental, basic, and hard to refute. Risks versus benefits are weighed, but ultimately, the patient makes the final decision. Doctors may refuse to treat if they believe the risks outweigh the benefits, but the patient is free to find another doctor who thinks otherwise. That's exactly what Erin Jones did when she called me on October 22, 2021.

Erin's husband Jason was a respected member of his community—sheriff's deputy, father of six, and loving husband. Prior to entering the hospital, he tried to get ivermectin to treat his COVID infection but was unable to find a doctor willing to prescribe it. He received no treatment in the week prior to entering the hospital, and like many, on day eight, his respiratory status declined to the point where he thought his life was in danger. He was admitted to Texas Health Huguley Hospital in Ft. Worth, Texas, on September 28, 2021.

He was not vaccinated and refused Remdesivir. Patients like Mr. Jones were labeled and treated differently. Mr. Jones's chart contained repeated documentation of "not vaccinated" and "refused Remdesivir," suggesting a negative bias from the medical staff. If he had been hospitalized with the flu, the admitting history and physical might have mentioned whether or not he received a flu shot, but it would not have been documented on a daily basis.

Mr. Jones's situation deteriorated, and he was put on a ventilator. After nearly a month, his doctors started to discuss hospice. His wife asked about ivermectin and was denied. Desperate to try anything that might save his life, she decided to sue the hospital and hired Ralph Lorigo and Beth Parlato as counsel.

Mrs. Jones texted me, "Well, when I talked to you that Friday, this dr [doctor] had told me that they were going to trach [perform a tracheostomy] him the early part of that next week. And if he didn't tolerate that, they would have a 'different' conversation with me.... Nurse said hospice. That's why I freaked out, got the attorneys and called you for the prescription."

Ralph and Beth, experts in medical litigation, gained prominence for suing 189 hospitals that denied dying patients access to ivermectin. They won half of these cases, and in those victories, all but three patients survived. Tragically, every patient in the cases they lost died. Notably, case outcomes strongly correlated with the political affiliation of the presiding judge. Republican judges ruled in favor of the patients, while Democrat judges sided with the hospitals. Consequently, patients' survival often hinged on the political leanings of the judge deciding their case.

Ralph and Beth had a well-tested strategy for all of their cases. They couldn't force the doctors in the hospital to give a medication, but if they could find a willing doctor, they could ask the judge to order the hospital to grant privileges to the doctor, and that doctor could administer the medication. They had used this approach with success in many previous cases. They just needed to find a doctor licensed in Texas who could help Mr. Jones.

That's where I came in. I was a member of FLCCC and was listed on their website as a doctor licensed in Texas. Erin scheduled a telemedicine appointment with me to discuss her husband's situation. She was fortunate the hospital allowed her to visit him daily, and she was very familiar with his medical condition. She knew which medications he was on and, as we texted frequently, was always aware of his vent settings. I often marveled at her diligence and dedication to help him. Somehow she managed to care for six children and still spend most of the day in the hospital with her husband.

My first response was to encourage her to transfer her husband to a hospital in Houston, United Memorial Medical Center (UMMC), where Dr. Joseph Varon was practicing. Dr. Varon is a critical care specialist and founding member of FLCCC who was a tireless warrior for inpatients during the pandemic. He had patients transported to him from all over the country—another medical phenomenon I'd never seen before, where critically ill patients were flown to other states because they couldn't get access to a once widely available generic medication. Dr. Varon is famous for working 715 continuous days without a break, admitting over 1,800 patients from all over the country. He had patients from California, Nebraska, Michigan, Rhode Island, Illinois, and Washington air transported to him for care. His mortality rate was 4.1 percent, while the rest of the country's was about 20 percent.

Once admitted to a hospital, you're in a very vulnerable position, especially if you don't have family there to advocate for you. Prior to the pandemic, most of us thought of the hospital as a place of safety. Now, one of the most common questions I get asked is if there is a hospital I trust. People have become quite fearful. Getting a second opinion while in a hospital is no easy task. Requesting transfer to another hospital is virtually impossible. It takes a massive amount of courage from the family to take the steps to transfer their sick family member, especially without having any background in medicine. The patient's family has to request the transfer, and doing so instantly puts the people taking care of the patient on defense. Typically, there are competing opinions amongst family members, and then the hospitals create obstacles. In the patients I tried to help, the hospitals' first response was to claim it was too dangerous to transfer the patient and put unnecessary fear in the family members. Often the hospital outright refused, despite not having the authority to do so.

Here's a typical example. In February 2022, I had a family in Oklahoma reach out to me about transferring their loved one from Integris Baptist Medical Center in Oklahoma to UMMC to be cared for by Dr. Varon.

From the family member, "The hospital is willing to transfer and assist. They cautioned there is a risk a mucous plug could come loose during transport with the movement." I had heard this before. I discussed it with Dr. Varon, who responded that the hospital was either trying to cover themselves for liability and/or to discourage transport, and he was not worried.

An hour later, the family member texted, "They are giving us a little trouble claiming Dr. Varon is not a critical care doctor. We are asking them to call again because we see he is chief of critical care at UMMC."

Dr. Varon was definitely a critical care doctor. An hour later, the family member texted back with hope. "Looks like they agreed now. They called UMMC and are waiting on a call back. Some progress!"

Two hours later, that hope was dashed. "I think they have been lying. The charge nurse is telling us now that they won't request it. They now say the other hospital has to do it. We are contacting lawyers to try to get legal help in the morning."

The sending hospital always initiates the transfer. The family was eventually able to transfer their loved one, but it took a lawyer to get it done.

Here's another example from the same time period, where a patient at Baylor Scott & White Medical Center—Grapevine in Texas required legal help in order to get transferred to Dr. Varon. I told the daughter, "Tell the hospital that you are transferring him. They will call UMMC and UMMC will call Dr. Varon to accept the transfer. The hospital should arrange transportation, but if they give you a hard time, Dr. Varon has an EMS connection that can help. They will give you excuses why he can't be transferred. Don't take no for an answer. Raise hell if you need to."

The daughter followed all the necessary steps, and the transfer seemed imminent. Then they were told their insurance company wouldn't allow it.

From the daughter:

> My mom hasn't heard back from Cigna. They have denied us access to dad. My mom was finally able to get back there but they said yesterday was a 'privilege' for both of us to be there. He's no longer on COVID protocol. Both of us ARE allowed to be there. They are punishing us because the transfer didn't go through. Dr. Reddy will NOT talk to mom, he sends his nurses in to do his dirty work.... Since the transfer didn't go through, they are punishing. They are not giving him the meds he needs and they are not lowering his oxygen. It's like they don't care and are punishing.

In the case of Jason Jones in Ft. Worth, Mrs. Jones decided to keep her husband at Texas Huguley, and based on what I was seeing when other people tried to transfer their loved ones, I understood why. Unlike most places, at Texas Huguley she was allowed to visit her husband every day.

At that time, I had treated 268 COVID patients with ivermectin and knew how safe it was, and I had no qualms about potential side effects if Mr. Jones were to take it. The only contraindication is pregnancy, but even pregnant women can take it if the potential benefit outweighs the risk. Mrs. Jones was familiar with the FLCCC's MATH+ protocol for hospitalized patients and asked if her husband could receive those medications as well. The plan was to sue the hospital, asking the court to grant me privileges so I could treat Mr. Jones with ivermectin and possibly the other medications.

I spoke with Mrs. Jones's attorney, Beth, about the strategy, and she asked that I provide a written prescription for the ivermectin that would be included in the legal documents. On November 2, 2021, I testified on behalf of Mrs. Jones, along with Senator Bob Hall from Texas State Senate District 2. The judge ruled in our favor, ordering Texas Huguley to grant me temporary emergency privileges with the stipulation that I was only allowed to administer ivermectin to Mr. Jones.

The judge ordered the hospital to make it happen within twenty-four hours, but instead the hospital set up immediate roadblocks. After I received the application, their credentialing person called me and said I also needed to submit two years of surgical case logs. I had recently gone through the credentialing process at Houston Methodist and had not had to do this. My case log history had no relevance to the purpose of the privileges I was granted by the court. The credentialing process was also universally streamlined during COVID so hospitals in need could have access to more physicians, but Texas Huguley ignored this. After completing an online application over twenty pages long, I sent them proof of my malpractice insurance, my DEA license information, my driver's license, list of surgeries, and two letters of reference. I somehow managed to get everything they needed by the following day, but the hospital stalled. Beth told me they were considering denying my privileges, which worried me because if you apply for privileges and are denied, it's considered a reportable event to the National Practitioner Data Bank (NPDB) and becomes a permanent mark on your record.

On November 3, 2021, Mrs. Jones texted me, "Do you know how hard it would be to get him to Houston where you could treat him? Or I am trying to get somewhere up here that you can treat him too. From what I understand the hospital is going to appeal the order from yesterday."

I responded, "What?!"

"Yes," she texted back. "They are going to fight the order. My only option is getting him out of here."

That Friday afternoon, November 5, 2021—three days after the court order telling the hospital to grant me temporary privileges—I received the following email from their administrator Tandra Cobern: "Dr. Bowden, I am notifying you that the Credentials Vice Chair, President of the Medical Staff and Department of Surgery Chair have all declined to grant you temporary privileges. We will continue to process your application in its entirety. This is not a denial of your application."

I forwarded it to Beth, who responded, "Apparently the doctors believe they are above a court order. They were ORDERED to grant you temporary privileges. It wasn't up for a discussion. They lost in Court."

The hospital had applied for a stay on the judge's order. That evening, the judge held a conference with the two parties. Another court order was filed on November 8, 2021, at 4:45 p.m. in our favor. The following day, on November 9, 2021—a week following the hearing and the original court order—I received a letter from Dr. Ronny Ford, the chief medical officer for Texas Huguley Hospital. He instructed me to reapply for privileges, explaining they would not accept my previous application and my reapplication was due by the end of the day. After consideration by the medical staff that evening, the application was going to the hospital's board of directors two days later. "If the Board approves your application" (ignoring the court order), then the hospital would allow me or my nurse to crush the ivermectin pills and flush them into Mr. Jones's feeding tube then immediately leave the hospital.

Beth instructed me to send a supplement to the application acknowledging everything Dr. Ford requested in this letter, but the hospital's attorney, Joshua Ross, said that wasn't enough and required me to complete the entire application over again. I also had to include the name and information for a nurse who would be administering the medication, as they were not willing to provide one from the hospital. In record time amidst a very busy clinic, I fulfilled the requirements and was assured by Beth that I was allowed to proceed.

The hospital appealed within thirty minutes of the judge signing the original order, but per Beth, they didn't get a stay on the order. Without a stay, I was legally permitted to administer the ivermectin. (A "stay" means that the original order is paused and cannot be acted on.) Beth was worried that, regardless of the order, the hospital would not let us in. The appeal hearing was a week away, meaning we had a week with the order in effect, and Mr. Jones could get a full week of ivermectin.

From Beth, "I'm going to send you the order from the court of appeals. The hospital didn't get their stay. That is amazing news for us! He can get the ivermectin so we have to figure this out with the nurse ASAP."

I responded, "I'm confused by the order!"

Beth said, "Hospital appealed to have our temporary order stayed. Appeals court didn't grant the stay. They granted moving up the appeal. So we have to have our appellate brief in by the next

Wednesday. That means the court will decide the appeal sometime after next Wednesday."

I asked, "So in the meantime he can get ivermectin?"

Beth responded, "So he can get one full week of ivermectin. Yes. I told Erin we need a nurse ASAP."

I was willing to fly to Dallas from Houston to administer it if needed, but given that he would require the medication administered daily, we scrambled to find a local nurse willing to do it. I posted the need for a nurse willing to administer ivermectin on my social media accounts, but Mrs. Jones had a connection. Her friend in Utah had a cousin who knew a willing nurse in Ft. Worth, Kimberley Witzel, and by the end of the day on November 10, we had that problem solved.

As required, I sent an email to Tandra at 5:15 p.m., forewarning her of the nurse's arrival. "Per the lawyers, everything is set. My nurse will arrive in about 30 minutes with the court order."

Kimberley showed up at 5:45 p.m. with Mr. Jones's wife. They were greeted by an administrator of the hospital and the charge nurse of the ICU, Jason Cain.

Erin texted me, "They said our order isn't valid."

Kimberley added, "They have a stay and waited til I got here. They've called the police on us."

I relayed the information to Beth, who said, "I told the charge nurse to call a deputy. There is no stay on the order."

I didn't know this at the time, but the hospital had sent a complaint to the Texas Medical Board about me, days after I initially spoke with Mr. Jones's wife and long before this incident even happened. Once the Board began their investigation, the hospital fattened their complaint with the claim Nurse Witzel caused a scene, but she recorded most of the incident, proving otherwise.

She texted me, "He [the cop] said hospital policy no recording. I argued that no patient info or HIPAA violation has occurred. He demanded I stop. I kept on for another minute til officer got loud with me, then I stopped n put phone away. Officer said, 'Since you stopped recording, u don't have to leave right this minute.' Jason [charge nurse] said 'actually I am requesting the nurse leave.' I gave Erin a hug, got up, and she walked me down. I cried when I got downstairs."

She added, "I was trying to be respectful to police since the one misunderstood who my attitude was toward. But it was very hard."

I was at my son's wrestling match when this was happening, and my phone died. Two hours later, I realized Mr. Jones never got the ivermectin, and the following day I learned that the hospital did have a stay on the order. The email notification from the appellate court had gone to Jerri Lynn Ward's spam folder, and Beth had no knowledge of it at the time. Jerri Lynn was the local attorney assisting in the case.

Prior to this, we had discussed whether or not to publicize what was happening. A reporter, Emily Miller, had been covering the story but keeping Mr. Jones's name private. On November 10, she texted me, "Do you want to see if the lawyer wants to make this stuff public? I've been hiding it for patient privacy but if it's open court, maybe the family will want more attention from the media to pressure the hospital? I just don't want to do anything to hurt their case."

Beth responded, "We always want the media to get a hold of the story if the hospital refuses to comply. Right now, they lost the stay on appeal and based on our conversations with atty [attorney], hospital will be complying. If they don't let you in when we finally have a nurse and you can get there for the first dose, then we need media to blow it up like we discussed yesterday."

Mrs. Jones first considered going public on November 7, texting me, "If I can't get answers... media may be my next option. Time is of the essence for Jason." On November 12, I told her I was going on *The Blaze* podcast with Daniel Horowitz and asked if I should publicize their names or keep them private. She said it was okay to publicize, then later that day we both did an interview with a local news station.

The hospital claimed I violated HIPAA by posting Mr. Jones's name on social media, despite documentation I provided from his wife, who was his medical power of attorney, that allowed me to publicize his name. Ironically, the hospital violated HIPAA by not redacting Mr. Jones's name and health information from the public court records.

A friend of Mrs. Jones set up a GoFundMe page to raise money for her legal bills. On November 17, they deleted her page without warning saying it violated their terms under their "Prohibited conduct" section. A GiveSendGo page was set up instead and is still active.

On November 11, 2021, the appellate court ruled in favor of Texas Huguley Hospital, and Mr. Jones was denied the opportunity to take ivermectin. The nurses took an extra step and tightly wrapped his feeding tube with a washcloth to prevent anyone from sneaking anything in.

His battle was far from over though. His wife had already been rubbing ivermectin on his feet and putting it under his tongue and a different doctor took over his care. He suffered repeated setbacks—recurrent pneumothoraces (lung collapse) requiring multiple chest tubes, sepsis, a gallbladder infection, and blood clots—but fought through and steadily improved.

On November 20, he opened his eyes and squeezed his wife's hand. Three days later, his wife, family, and friends held a rally to raise awareness about Jason's treatment at Texas Huguley. On November 29, he was weaned off Precedex, a sedative used for anxiety in the ICU that has the unfortunate side effect of lowering blood pressure, sometimes requiring additional medications to bring it back up. Mrs. Jones held another rally on December 7, and on December 10, he was able to tell his wife he loved her.

Erin debated about transferring him to Dr. Varon at UMMC in Houston or the rehab hospital Kindred in Ft. Worth. She had heard bad things about Kindred, but Dr. Varon was more optimistic and said he would get good physical therapy there. She decided on Kindred, and he was transferred on January 1, 2022. Erin texted me:

> Even though he has the same doctor, this place is more aggressive getting people off the ventilator. He did have to go back on the sedation some because of the sepsis. His body was so tired fighting the infections. I think starting tomorrow, they will really work with him. It makes a huge difference with them here saying that they want him off the ventilator compared to Huguley saying they are just support care. So not much chance for getting 'alternative' medicine, but hopefully more aggressive for healing him.

I told Erin, "He's the toughest patient I've ever seen." He sat in a chair for the first time on January 26. He was weaned off the ventilator in early February, was moved out of the ICU in mid-February, and in mid-March, passed his swallow test and was able to drink liquids and eat soft food. On March 28, they removed his chest tube, and two days later, his PEG tube (feeding tube). On April 22, 2022, he was allowed outside to celebrate his son Jacob's eighteenth birthday—the first time outside in seven months. He was finally released on May 18, 2022, nearly six months after being admitted. He had lost half his body weight, starting at 240 lbs. and leaving at 120 lbs.

Erin and I texted regularly, and I was always impressed with her grasp of the details of her husband's condition. She sent me his medications, vital signs, and ventilator settings and sent me photos and videos. As things settled down, we texted less frequently, but in late February 2023, she sent me an unfortunate update. "We have had a tough couple of months. It's like we hit a wall in December. He didn't really need any medical care ... then bam. We were actually admitted into CCU [critical care unit] this morning. This has made the 3rd hospital stay since December. I'm just praying we can get through this and back on the upswing of things." At that point, his weight was down to 105 lbs. He fought back hard and managed to get out of the ICU, but on April 10th, Erin texted me that he was in hospice. The following day—April 11, 2023—he passed.

Mr. Jones's experience was somewhat miraculous in that he survived a very prolonged hospital stay, but tragically he should have never ended up in the hospital to begin with. Had he received early treatment, I am certain he would not have been hospitalized, and even after hospitalization, he most likely would have survived with proper treatment. His wife Erin has told me she has regrets, wishing she had done more, but I honestly don't know anyone who fought as hard as she did for her husband. The entirety of the blame rests on the doctors who refused to treat him, the hospital administrators that fought tooth and nail to deny him access to an incredibly safe medication, and ultimately, the FDA that demonized ivermectin to the point that most doctors wouldn't consider using it.

Jason Jones and his family lost their legal battle in the fall of 2021, but I was not done fighting. A year later, on November 1, 2022, I drove to the Galveston United States Post Office and Courthouse, with the United States District Court for the Southern District of Texas, to attend the first hearing of *Apter, Bowden, and Marik v. FDA*.

CHAPTER 7

Turning Point

Early November of 2021, during the third and largest surge of the pandemic, was a turning point in my career. COVID vaccine mandates started in Houston in April 2021, and by September, they had spread nationally. Meanwhile, I was observing the failure of the shots to prevent transmission and lower severity while observing the success of early treatment. I had very sick patients scared to go to the hospital, and I had people who were not my patients pleading with me to help them or their loved ones escape from hospitals. At that point, the festering doubts I had about the government's intentions were solidified, and all trust was gone.

Three events occurred on a single day that brought everything to a head. Had they been spaced out, even days apart, the outcome would have likely been different. But at the conclusion of a very stressful week, I received three bits of bad news that prompted me to make a decision.

On November 6, 2021, I sent this email to my patients and posted it on my website:

Dear BreatheMD Community,

Yesterday was a turning point for me as a physician. Earlier this week, I testified on behalf of a dying father of 6 who was being refused ivermectin by his treating physicians. The judge ruled in our favor, telling the hospital's lawyer that I was to be granted temporary privileges and allowed to administer medications to my patient. I have never been denied privileges and have never been sued. My professional record is spotless with no grounds to not grant me privileges, but yesterday afternoon, Texas Huguley Hospital in Ft. Worth, TX informed me that my request for privileges was denied.

I then received a call from a patient with a history of bladder cancer who was looking for a new urologist. Her current urologist works for Methodist Hospital. He called her to tell her that Methodist was discussing denying care for unvaccinated people, and she should start looking for a urologist who can see her.

The final straw was the email I received from one of the surgery centers I operate at. I was informed that in order to keep operating there, myself and my patients would need to provide proof of vaccination. I kindly told them that was not going to work for me, and I would operate elsewhere.

Given the current climate and the writing on the wall, I am shifting my practice focus to treating the unvaccinated. In order to make room for the unvaccinated who cannot find care, I will not be accepting new patients with routine ENT problems who are vaccinated. I will continue to care for established patients, vaccinated or not, and would never turn anyone away with a life-threatening illness based on their vaccination status. But this is my way of taking a stand, and I hope other physicians will follow.

I am not anti-vaccination, but all the data I have collected suggests that the vaccine is not working. 42% of the patients we treated last month with IV monoclonal antibodies for symptomatic COVID-19 were fully vaccinated. I believe vaccination is a personal choice and like everything else in medicine, should be protected by HIPAA. I understand this alienates many of you, but all my opinions are based on my clinical experience and not the news.

Thank you for your understanding.

Best,

Mary Talley Bowden MD

The email struck a nerve and was shared far and wide. A reporter from the *Houston Chronicle*, Julian Gill, reached out to me for comment. I texted him this statement: "I've cared for well over a thousand people with COVID-19, and I want everyone to receive treatment. Moving forward, I will only accept NEW patients who are unvaccinated because they are being marginalized. I am simply doing what I can to restore their power and make sure they have medical care." Julian, of course, did not publish this.

News of the email spread to California, where a social media influencer who claims to practice obstetrics, Dr. Jen Gunter (author of the website The Vajenda), encouraged the public to report me to the Texas Medical Board. "Many hospitals require board certification for privileges and many insurers also require it. Just step up and do the right thing."

The same day, another obstetrician with over a million followers on YouTube, Mama Doctor Jones, posted a highly derogatory video painting me as an anti-vax grifter. "I made an informercial [sic] to advertise Dr. Mary Bowden's anti-vaxx practice." The video went viral on TikTok.

A physician posted the Mama Doctor Jones video on the private Facebook group Houston Women's Physicians Group. Like a scene from the movie *Mean Girls,* the women celebrated the video with glee while calling me names. Dr. Nelly Arielle Heiman, an obstetrician at Houston Methodist, wrote, "I'm just going to say it because I know the majority of people in this group will agree—we do not support you. You are providing misinformation and supporting harmful treatments. You are adding fuel to the fire. There is nothing you can say that will change our minds so just go find a different FB (Facebook) group."

I responded, "Given that there are over 2000 doctors in this group and your post got 4 likes, I suspect there are people on here that don't agree with the witch hunt you all are launching. But no one would dare speak up given how brutally viciously you are attacking me. I am putting myself on the line to stand up against vaccine mandates and you are trying to ruin me. I have plenty of supporters outside of this group, including hundreds of very grateful patients."

One of my patients forwarded my controversial email to her friend Emily Miller, a reporter in Washington, DC, who had once worked at the FDA. Emily reached out to me and ran a story on my email followed by a series of stories on Jason Jones. Along with Michael Berry, she was the first reporter to try to legitimize my voice, and we still communicate regularly.

I drew a line in the sand on November 6, and the following day, Sunday, November 7, I doubled down, posting, "Vaccine mandates are wrong" twenty-five times on Twitter with twenty-five different screenshots of comments from patients responding to my email. I had very few followers at the time, and the posts only had a few likes … but the move did not go unnoticed.

That evening, at 9 p.m., Mas, the ENT I was doing research with at Houston Methodist, sent me the following email. "Hi Mary Talley, I had a friend tell me that you had mentioned that HMH was discussing not providing patient care for those that are unvaccinated. I can tell you that that is unconditionally false. HMH as well as my department will always take care of any patient, vaccinated or not. Can you please correct that in any information that you give out?"

I responded, "Heard it from a patient of mine who has no reason to lie. I will not correct the truth."

He replied:

My department will always care for any patient, vaccinated or not. As a member of HMH Med Exec committee and I can tell you there has not been any discussions about this at HMH at the leadership level. That is the truth. Why would I have any reason to lie to you? Could it not be conceivable that her urologist, who is not in a leadership position, is incorrect? You would rather believe third hand information and propagate your patient's statement without verifying the source?

I responded, "It is very consistent with what patients are telling me. They are scared to tell their doctors they aren't vaccinated and report being treated by lepers by hospital staff and doctors. I wrote exactly what the patient told me and I'm not retracting it."

He said, "Why take their word instead of mine?"

I answered, "I believe that you would take care of an unvaccinated person, and one of your patients actually asked me if she should be worried and I said no. I absolutely believe that my patient's urologist said what she told me he said. Why are you so certain he didn't? You don't even know who it was."

Mas responded, "I am not saying that the urologist didn't say that. I said the urologist may have given out misinformation that is not correct. All I am asking is please verify your sources before posting."

"Seems highly unlikely that the urologist would misinterpret what was being discussed in staff meetings and then call the patient to tell her," I wrote.

He said, "Maybe reach out to the urologist to confirm? That way you will know for sure."

I concluded, "Why is this such a big deal to you and to Methodist? If it's not true, then there's nothing to worry about. I'm one little doctor in a massive system."

The following day, in the spirit of full transparency, I sent another email to my patients, where I included what Mas had told me, specifically that Houston Methodist does not have a policy in place to deny care to unvaccinated patients. While writing this book, I discovered that Square, the platform I used to send this, erased all my emails as well as the responses from patients between November 5, 2021, and November 21, 2021, and I have not been able to recover them.

One of the doctors from the Houston Women's Physicians Facebook Group reported this email and some of my social media posts to Houston Methodist, claiming I was spreading misinformation, telling pregnant women to take ivermectin, and violating HIPAA.

Other than the email exchange I had with Mas on November 7, I had no idea what was brewing at Methodist and continued to fight for Jason Jones.

November 10 was the day Jason Jones was supposed to get ivermectin for the first time. But when the hospital refused entry to my nurse, we decided to go public. This was a shared decision with Erin Jones, his wife; Beth Parlato, Erin's attorney; and Emily Miller, the journalist who had been covering the story. The purpose was to pressure the hospital to follow the court order.

That same day, the group No License for Disinformation (NLFD) attacked me online, posting on Twitter all the necessary information for anyone in the world to report me to the Texas Medical Board. NLFD no longer exists, but it was led by California emergency room doctor Nick Sawyer.

> We are building a coalition of physicians, nurses, allied health professionals, disability advocates, parents, and concerned citizens who understand the threat and consequences of this dangerous disinformation and empowering them to speak out against physicians who abuse their status and platforms to spread disinformation, and speak up and call on the medical boards to hold these physicians accountable according to existing consumer protection laws and state statutes.[1]

Dr. Sawyer's mission was to silence doctors by threatening the licenses of physicians he believed were spreading COVID misinformation.

Methodist ignored the follow-up email I sent to my patients stating it does not have a policy to deny care to the unvaccinated. The next day, on Friday afternoon at 4:30 p.m., November 12, 2021, I received a text message from Julian Gill, a reporter at the *Houston Chronicle*.

"Hi Dr. Bowden, I'm told you've been suspended from Houston Methodist pending further investigation because of your comments on social media. I plan to report that this afternoon but wanted to give you an opportunity to comment."

I was stunned. "No! News to me. I have not received any notification like that. Who told you that?!"

He responded, "A source at the hospital informed me but I will clarify if that's true with their media team before reporting anything. I can hold the story until 6:30 this evening to give you time to respond. Please send me any updated statements you would like me to include by then."

I responded, "All I did was report the takeaways from the Global COVID summit. FAR different from telling patients not to get vaccinated. I have a lawyer helping me with defamation so please take care not to misconstrue the information."

He said, "The information you've shared about COVID in your email and on social media is misleading and we are reporting it as such."

I answered, "Well just be careful what you say because I do have a lawyer. Methodist pays you to advertise correct?"

Julian said, "Understood. Please let me know if you have any further comment on your suspension or the reasons cited by the hospital."

I texted him, "All of my comments are backed by clinical experience. I have been open 7 days a week since the pandemic began, performing over 80,000 COVID tests and treated over 2000 patients with COVID. These facts should be included. Else the story is not complete. And hence is misleading."

After the exchange, I went to Twitter and saw that Houston Methodist had posted a five-part thread about me:

> Dr. Mary Bowden, who recently joined the medical staff at Houston Methodist Hospital, is using her social media accounts to express her personal and political opinions about the COVID-19 vaccine and treatments. (1/5)
>
> These opinions, which are harmful to the community, do not reflect reliable medical evidence or the values of Houston Methodist, where we have treated more than 25,000 COVID-19 inpatients, and where all our employees and physicians are vaccinated to protect our patients. (2/5)
>
> Despite what she has posted, Houston Methodist does not and will never deny care to a patient based on vaccination status. (3/5)
>
> Dr. Bowden, who has never admitted a patient at Houston Methodist Hospital, is

> spreading dangerous misinformation which is not based in science. (4/5)
>
> Furthermore, Dr. Bowden has told Houston Methodist that she is vaccinated, as required of all physicians who practice at Houston Methodist. (5/5)[2]

I then checked my email and found confirmation—Methodist had suspended my privileges for thirty days.

The following day, Winnie Brown, director of medical staff services, sent out an email on behalf of Dr. Stuart Solomon to the entire medical staff, over thirty thousand people, condemning me.

> Dear Colleagues,
>
> Many of you have expressed concern about Dr. Mary Bowden's now public opinions about COVID-19 vaccines and treatments, and the misinformation she is spreading about hospitals not treating the unvaccinated. This behavior by Bowden, who has provisional privileges at Houston Methodist Hospital, will not be tolerated. Each of us is entitled to our own political, social and religious beliefs. I CARE is the cornerstone of all of our professional existence and a direct attack on it will not be tolerated at any level.
>
> I am sharing with you the official response from HM about this situation:
>
> Dr. Mary Bowden, who recently joined the medical staff at Houston Methodist Hospital, is using her social media accounts to express her personal and political opinions about the COVID-19 vaccine and treatments. These opinions, which are harmful to the community, do not reflect reliable medical evidence or the values of Houston Methodist, where we have treated more than 25,000 COVID-19 inpatients, and where all our employees and physicians are vaccinated to

protect our patients. Despite what she has posted, Houston Methodist does not and will never deny care to a patient based on vaccination status.

Dr. Bowden, who has never admitted a patient at Houston Methodist Hospital, is spreading dangerous misinformation which is not based in science. Furthermore, Dr. Bowden attested, as of June 6, 2021, to Houston Methodist that she is vaccinated—a necessary requisite for continued medical staff membership.

As usual, I am available for your questions or concerns.

Stuart L. Solomon, M.D.

Medical Staff President

Part of my soul died that afternoon. The years of training, the immense commitment I made to a profession, the pride of doing something that truly helps people—it all felt meaningless, and I questioned why I had bothered going into medicine. I holed away in my house that weekend, agonizing over what had happened and hiding from the world, but to no avail. The media hunted me down and found me. Three hours following the tweets, I received a text message from a reporter at ABC13, Jessica Willey, asking for an interview or a statement. Like Julian Gill, I have no idea how she got my cell phone number but can only presume Houston Methodist provided it to both of them. I also heard from Bill Barajas, a reporter from KPRC 2 in Houston, who asked me to do an interview. Because I knew him (he reported on our clinic doing a study comparing saliva testing to nasal swab testing for COVID), I agreed. I wanted my side of the story out there.

I have purposely avoided rewatching that interview; I viewed it for the second and last time just moments before writing this paragraph, and I don't care to ever watch it again. If I search my name on YouTube or Google, this interview always appears... a glaring reminder of my lowest point during this saga. The thumbnail is impossible to miss; purposely chosen to paint me in a negative light, I look like I just crawled out of bed and am reaching for the bottle. I did the interview from my bedroom over Zoom. My eyes never looked at the camera and were incredibly puffy from crying. I bet Bill was thrilled; at the end, I nearly broke down in tears.

To say I was overwhelmed was an understatement. The following day, Keith Allen from CNN reached out, followed by CBS, NBC, the *Washington Post*—the requests kept coming. By Monday morning, all major national news stations and newspapers were reporting the story. A year later, I would meet a psychologist from Great Britain who told me he heard the news across the pond. I had people from all over the world reaching out. Navigating uncharted territory, I had to choose a path.

CHAPTER 8

Going on Offense

The media blitz left me in a state of shock, but I had enough sense to find an attorney. A friend referred me to Steve Mitby, a highly experienced trial lawyer in Houston.

I told Steve I wanted to resign from Houston Methodist right away, but being that it was the weekend, he counseled I was unlikely to get a response. We aimed for Monday. In the meantime, he helped me draft a resignation letter and prepare a statement for the incoming wave of media requests.

My experience with the media was limited, so I turned to radio show host Michael Berry for help. Michael connected me with Wayne Dolcefino. Wayne is an Emmy award-winning investigative reporter, known and feared far and wide for his mastery at exposing people and institutions that abuse their power. While I licked my wounds, Wayne and my attorney Steve planned our offense.

Monday morning was a fresh start. I sent my resignation letter to Houston Methodist and held a press conference outside my office. I was sick with some other non-COVID virus that caused me to have laryngitis. Running on adrenaline, I had a busy clinic schedule that I paused to squeeze in the press conference. Wayne prepared talking points and, like a coach in the locker room, tried to convince me I was worthy. I attempted to focus on what Wayne wanted me to say, but I was too frazzled to memorize anything. Minutes before heading out my office door to face a sea of cameras, I spoke to Michael Berry. I can't remember the details, but whatever he said gave me enough confidence to walk out the door.

Looking back, I'm proud of myself—and a bit surprised. If things hadn't been moving so quickly, I'm pretty sure I would never have done a press conference. I have always disliked public speaking and still do. But now, before stepping up to a podium, I recall how difficult that press conference was and hold my shoulders a little higher.

The video of the press conference went viral and, to date, has five million views on KPRC 2's YouTube channel. KPRC 2 turned off the comments, so I'm uncertain how the jury weighed in, but the journalist who covered it, Bill Barajas, was promoted to evening news anchor.

During the press conference, I spoke of my successful track record in treating COVID patients, the breakthrough cases I was seeing, and my right to publicly report my clinical opinion. I spoke of how I deeply researched the safety of ivermectin before prescribing it. And I reiterated my condemnation of vaccine mandates.

Of all the points I made during the press conference, the one that felt most important was the complete lack of transparency from Houston Methodist. As the first hospital to mandate the COVID shots, Houston Methodist Hospital was well-equipped to collect and analyze data on their safety and efficacy. No surprise, the hospital was—and still is—silent on the matter.

I believe Houston Methodist did not volunteer, but was chosen, to be the first major employer in the country to mandate the shots.

The federal government knew if they could get away with mandates in the seemingly red state of Texas, they could get away with them anywhere. A year after instituting the mandate, the hospital received an anonymous $50 million donation, perhaps a reward for its efforts.

I suspect that if the COVID vaccine outcomes had supported Houston Methodist's agenda, the hospital would have widely publicized their data. Instead, I exposed the shot's lack of efficacy and the ethical issues with the mandates. Unable to counter my claims with data, the hospital resorted to publicly humiliating me, aiming to silence me and warn other physicians of the consequences of dissent.

This public shaming echoed the "struggle sessions" of China's Cultural Revolution, where "class enemies" faced verbal and physical abuse in workplaces, classrooms, or auditoriums. Today, such tactics are amplified online, where social media's vast reach makes modern struggle sessions far more impactful. Houston Methodist's announcements on Twitter and to the *Houston Chronicle* launched a highly effective digital struggle session against me. Their actions were amplified by mainstream media and social media influencers around the world, and I received thousands of hate messages. One I won't forget came from a professor of neurosurgery at the University of Pennsylvania whom I have never met. Dr. David O'Rourke took time out of his busy schedule to email me, "Stop the online bullshit you quack—only seeing unvaccinated patients? You should lose your license promptly before spreading more misinformation." Locally, the *Houston Chronicle* featured me in their New Year's edition as one of the most controversial Houstonians of 2021, and Harris County Judge Lina Hidalgo tweeted I was a conspiracy theorist.

For a long time, I felt very self-conscious around Houston, only finding relief when I left the city. I avoided eye contact at the grocery store, sat in the corner at my children's sports events, and saw my social life evaporate. Even rare invitations were declined. Faced with threatening voicemails and an incident where a man stormed into my office, I feared for my safety.

The humiliation I endured still lingers, but, as my dad likes to say, they stepped on the wrong hornet. The hospital launched their attack on a Friday afternoon, and by Monday, I had mounted a strong counterattack. Four years later, my resolve remains unwavering, and my voice has grown exponentially. Last month, I was interviewed by both Tucker Carlson and Joe Rogan. The Texas legislature recently passed a resolution to honor my work during the pandemic, and *Texas Scorecard* presented me with the 2023 Conservative Leader Award, complete with an engraved sword that now proudly hangs on my bedroom wall. Today, I walk into the grocery store with confidence and am warmly greeted by other parents at my children's school.

I had many choices during the pandemic. I could have shut my doors. I could have chosen not to treat. I could have kept quiet. And when Methodist attacked, I could have retreated, closed my office, and gone back to being a full-time mother. But I didn't. I've always been one to stand up for myself, perhaps because I grew up with two older brothers, but my first and only instinct was to fight back.

The hospital did not succeed in silencing me, but their actions had a ripple effect, sending a loud and clear message to other physicians about the consequences of challenging their dogma. Though other physicians affiliated with Houston Methodist quit over the mandates, and a few even sued, no other physicians spoke out against them like I did, nor have any paid the same price in doing so.

CHAPTER 9

Canceled

Though many people reached out to encourage me following the press conference, my professional circles quickly unraveled. Houston Methodist's actions created a chain reaction, and I was canceled from multiple organizations, kicked off the board of the Validation Institute, removed from accessing the American Board of Otolaryngology's (ABO-HNS) online group forum, and quietly forced out of my leadership positions with FMMA and the Direct Specialty Care Alliance Board. One group, the Texas Medical Association, not only shunned me, but actively campaigned against me.

FMMA, Free Market Medical Association, is a group I passionately supported prior to the pandemic. As a specialist starting a cash-only practice, I was entering unfamiliar territory and thirsty for guidance. I became active on LinkedIn looking for other doctors doing what I was doing and stumbled upon FMMA. The group embodies exactly what I was striving to accomplish—practice medicine free from the shackles of third parties (insurance companies, hospitals, and the government) and provide transparent pricing to my patients. I also connected with Houston radiologist Dr. Cristin Dickerson who runs an innovative company, Green Imaging. With a footprint all over the country, Green Imaging connects patients with radiology centers offering affordable cash pricing. Cristin is also very active with FMMA, heading their Houston chapter.

Cristin was kind enough to meet with me and give advice, but after our meeting, I realized her strategy was different from mine. Cristin's company is large and contracts with multiple third parties—not insurance companies but third-party administrators (TPAs). There are many types of TPAs, and free market physicians are more likely to work with a TPA who represents businesses that self-fund their health plan. Generally, TPAs are easier to work with than insurance companies, but they still serve as a middleman between patients and doctors. I was aiming to avoid any sort of middleman. In my opinion, contracting with TPAs was just a more palatable way to stick corporate interests between the doctor-patient relationship.

Despite having different approaches, Cristin and I kept in touch, and she invited me to join her Vistage group. In late June 2021, as COVID started to surge for the third time and in the wake of the Houston Methodist shot mandates, Cristin asked me to become coleader of the Houston chapter of FMMA with her and Dr. Juliet Breeze.

Cristin and I never discussed our views on COVID, but I sensed we were not on the same page when she started attending all our Vistage meetings over Zoom. On the surface, we were collegial, but her claws came out on social media, where she joined other doctors on Facebook and LinkedIn criticizing me. Though she was certainly allowed to disagree with me, I felt her doing so publicly—given that we were in the same Vistage group and were supposed to support each other—was crossing a line.

After the leader of our Vistage group confronted Cristin about attacking me online, she decided to leave the group. I knew other members shared similar views as Cristin regarding the pandemic and how I was handling it, so I also decided to drop out. Dues were expensive, and I didn't want to pay money and carve out valuable time to spend with people who were silently judging me.

At the same time, I was quietly kicked out of my leadership position at FMMA. Our last meeting was November 4, 2021, and a week later, following the news coverage with Methodist on November 12, I was removed from all further email communications. Dr. Juliet Breeze, the other coleader, had a contract with Methodist during the pandemic to administer monoclonal antibodies at her urgent care clinics. We were like-minded about making healthcare more affordable and transparent but not about bodily autonomy and informed consent. Cristin and Juliet didn't bother to tell me I was no longer a leader; rather, Cristin told the national leaders I was too busy to participate and then stopped including me in emails. When I discovered what had happened and brought this to the FMMA's attention, I was disappointed the leaders did nothing.

In a similar fashion, I was removed from both the advisory board for the Validation Institute, an organization supporting price transparency in healthcare, and the Direct Specialty Care Alliance, a group I helped form with the goal of bringing together independent specialists. Neither institution had the courage to tell me I was no longer on the board. Instead, they just dropped me from all further email communications.

Rather than nudge me out, one organization went on offense. I've been a member of the Texas Medical Association (TMA) since 2003, and though never actively involved, I perceived the organization as an ally, giving solo doctors like myself a voice. Membership, with dues of over $800 a year, is required if using Texas Medical Liability Trust (TMLT) for malpractice insurance, as I do. This requirement never bothered me, until I unsuccessfully tried to switch insurance carriers. TMLT has a virtual monopoly in Texas, so I have no choice but to pay dues to an organization I now know is trying to take my license away.

As the largest state medical organization in the country, TMA was once pro-doctor and pro-patient—a protector of the little guys against insurance companies and the government. But as evidenced by what happened during the pandemic, TMA is now merely an extension of government public health agencies. In recent years, TMA has lobbied for both medical mandates and physician censorship. The group opposed both the COVID-19 Vaccine Freedom Act and SB 14, a bill prohibiting medical and surgical modification of gender in minors. After a prolonged battle, both bills passed, but in the most conservative state in the country, TMA vehemently opposed two laws protecting patient autonomy and informed consent.

Through the COVID-19 Community Corps, the federal government created financial incentives for organizations like TMA to target and deplatform individual citizens online and mass report doctors and nurses to licensing boards. COVID-19 Community Corps started with 275 founding members and grew to over fifteen thousand members by 2023. The web of financial distributions is too vast to trace, but a few of those organizations and influencers directly crossed my path. In addition to No License for Disinformation and the social media influencers Mama Doctor Jones and Jen Gunter (the Vajenda), Shots Heard Round the World was another group that launched an online attack against me, encouraging the public to report me to the Texas Medical Board. Led by pediatrician Dr. Todd Wolynn and administrator Chad Hermann, the group describes themselves as a "rapid-response digital cavalry,"[1] providing members with suggestions on whom to pursue online and how to do it. An ally of mine managed to infiltrate the group and gain access to their membership roster. I was shocked to discover Texas Medical Association was on their membership list.

In recent years, the online assault has quieted down, but my most ardent online opponent, former pharmacist turned social media influencer Savannah Sparks, has continued her assault since sinking her teeth into me over four years ago. Going by "RxOrcist," Savannah has a large following of toxic followers on TikTok and created multiple viral videos intended to incite her angry army against me. Her loyal delegates left a slew of nasty reviews on Google about me and sent hate emails and threatening phone messages to my office. Savannah's sole purpose is to target people she disagrees with and try to ruin their lives. Many of her other victims have reached out to me seeking support. I reported her to the FBI for online harassment and intended to sue her for defamation, but my attorney suffered a stroke right before filing the suit. My plate has been too full to pursue her further, and given that my online army, at least on X, far exceeds hers at this point, I've decided to just ignore her.

From a professional standpoint, the most disappointing setback was getting canceled from the ABO-HNS online forum, a group I participated in often and highly valued as a source to bounce off complex clinical questions with colleagues. When COVID hit, I was relatively quiet on the forum and purposely avoided bringing up any controversy, but when my views made national news, two ENTs, Dr. Oscar Tamez and Dr. Robert McLean, wrote posts applauding my stance. I replied, "Thank you Dr. McLean for sharing this. I hope more physicians will speak up. Silence is compliance and what is happening is frightening." That was the extent of my controversial comments, but for that, the moderators kicked me off.

I was only able to read a few responses before losing access. One doctor, David Roberson, made a lengthy argument as to why I was not suited to treat COVID patients, claiming I needed to treat thousands of patients before I would be ready. His argument might have made sense under normal circumstances, but it failed to take into account the fact that we were dealing with a novel disease during a public health emergency. And though I had not treated thousands of patients at that point, my ENT practice did transform into a full-time COVID clinic. By the time the pandemic was over, I had treated more patients with COVID than I had ever treated any other disease. I became more than an expert.

No one received training on how to treat COVID. The "standard of care" was created by government doctors with no firsthand experience treating COVID. Typically, standard of care is a passive backstop used as a defense when things go wrong, but during the pandemic, it morphed into an offensive weapon used to take down any doctor who didn't comply with government mandates. For the first time in my career, I had to choose between following the standard of care and what I believed was in the best interest of my patients. Whereas most doctors chose the standard of care, I chose my patients. Like many other doctors during this time—Drs. Mollie James, Richard Edgerly, Joe Varon, Peter McCullough, Pierre Kory, Kirk Moore, Ben Marble, Paul Marik, Meryl Nass, Theresa Long, Kirk Milhoan, Simone Gold, Angie Farella, Steve LaTulippe, Charles Hoffe, Sherri Tenpenny, Ryan Cole, Scott Jensen, James Thorp, Molly Rutherford, Renata Moon, Kelly Victory, Richard Urso, Sam Sigoloff, Stella Immanuel, Michael Turner, Eric Hensen, Richard Bartlett, Scott Miller, Ron Creque, and many others—the establishment did everything they could to destroy physicians who questioned their definition of standard of care. All of us on this list have had to defend our licenses to our state medical board.

I never got to respond to Dr. Roberson. With no opportunity to defend myself, I was electronically erased—the first of many times to come.

CHAPTER 10

Reported

Following the online struggle session, Houston Methodist Hospital continued their attack by reporting me to both the Texas Medical Board and the National Practitioner Data Bank (NPDB), claiming I resigned while under investigation. Reports to the NPDB are serious, typically permanent, and used by hospitals to deny privileges.

The purpose of this rule is to prevent physicians from fleeing the scene of a crime. If a physician commits blatant malpractice and the hospital investigates, the threat of being reported to NPDB serves to cement the physician in place until the investigation is complete. My situation, however, was unique, as patient care was not part of the reason for the investigation. As defined in their own bylaws, Houston Methodist Hospital may only launch an investigation if the issue involves patient care. The hospital publicly declared they suspended my privileges for spreading "dangerous misinformation" and correctly stated I had never admitted a patient to their hospital. Unfortunately, this subtle but significant fact was completely ignored by the Texas Medical Board, and I still have a mark on my record from the National Practitioner Data Bank.

In addition to claiming I resigned privileges while being under investigation, TMB initially alleged I violated HIPAA, prescribed a dangerous drug (ivermectin) without a physician-patient relationship, failed to supervise, and sent a nurse to Texas Huguley Hospital to administer ivermectin to a patient without having privileges at the hospital. Without facts to back up these claims, all were eventually dropped but for the last one.

My social media activity has played a large part in TMB's pursuit. TMB alleged I advised pregnant patients to take ivermectin, citing my response to a tweet by Mama Doctor Jones about pregnant women dying from COVID, where I commented, "Should have tried ivermectin." I explained to the Board that I never prescribed ivermectin to pregnant women, clarified that my tweet was directed at a fellow physician, and noted that ivermectin, while a Pregnancy Category C drug, can be used if a physician determines the benefits outweigh the risks. In a life-and-death situation, suggesting ivermectin could be considered reasonable.

TMB further claimed I violated HIPAA by going public about Jason Jones, the patient at Texas Huguley Hospital whom I tried to help get ivermectin. I was very sensitive to the wishes of his wife and legal proxy and didn't go public until she gave me permission to do so. I have her permission documented. Notably, we discovered that Texas Huguley Hospital's attorneys breached HIPAA by failing to redact Mr. Jones's personal information from public court records.

The initial hearing (informal settlement conference or ISC) was scheduled for July 2022 then postponed until February 2023. This hearing—like all future interactions I would have with the Board—occurred over Zoom rather than in person, presumably due to persistent fears of contagion. Two members of the Board, a physician and a nonphysician, presided over the hearing along with their lawyers.

Through FOIA requests, I discovered that Texas Medical Board members were well-acquainted with me and my case prior to the informal settlement conference. On November 17, 2021, nonphysician board member Sharon Barnes emailed a highly critical *Houston Chronicle* article targeting me to other Board members and Jarrett Schneider, head of media relations. Around the same time, Barnes also participated in a group text with two other Board members discussing my case.

At an ISC, an anonymous expert reviews allegations and submits written recommendations. The Board is required to investigate complaints before proceeding, but depositions revealed they accepted the hospital's claims without contacting my witnesses. The anonymous expert provides only written testimony, with no opportunity for cross-examination. All ISC meeting records are sealed and cannot be shared publicly.

The panel proposed a settlement: a $5,000 fine, eight hours of continuing medical education (CME), and retaking the jurisprudence exam—a medical-legal test all Texas physicians must pass for licensure, which I had passed years earlier. Stunned, my attorneys had no chance to advise me before I outright rejected the offer. Feeling as if I had been punched in the gut, I used what little breath I could muster to loudly declare, "I do not accept your proposal."

Though I do not regret rejecting their offer, I did not anticipate the consequences of refusing to bend a knee. As I write this now, almost four years and $260,000 in legal fees later, I am still trying to clear my name. Following my refusal to accept their offer, on April 25, 2023, the Board filed a formal complaint against me in the State Office of Administrative Hearings (SOAH). This is an administrative court, run by the executive branch, and solely funded by the sixty state agencies SOAH oversees. The process is similar to a judicial proceeding with evidence, hearings, motions, and orders, but after the ALJ (administrative law judge) makes a recommendation, the power is handed back to the agency. The agency makes the final decision on determination of guilt and subsequent punishment against the defendant.

Historically, administrative courts have favored state agencies, influenced by the 1984 Supreme Court case *Chevron U.S.A., Inc. v. Natural Resources Defense Council, Inc.* This case set a precedent allowing federal agencies to win most cases (60 to 90 percent) by giving reasonable agencies the benefit of the doubt when interpreting unclear laws. Critics argued this gave agencies excessive power, and this eventually led to the 2024 Supreme Court's *Loper Bright (Loper Bright Enterprises v. Raimondo)* decision ending *Chevron.* Now, instead of automatically deferring to government agencies' interpretations, courts must independently determine the meaning of ambiguous statutes, shifting more interpretive power to judges. This change makes it tougher for agencies to win.

While *Chevron* deference was overturned by the Supreme Court, Texas still grants courts the ability to defer to an agency's reasonable interpretation of an ambiguous statute. Unlike *Chevron,* however, Texas's approach is narrower, requiring formal proceedings for deference. Regardless, deference laws do not apply during State Office of Administrative Hearings proceedings. When I appeal, my case will reach the state courts where these laws will apply.

SOAH processes an average of twenty-five thousand complaints per year, and the majority are completed within eight months. My case has dragged on far longer, with two settlement offers, three amended complaints, two continuances, failed mediation, and twenty-six orders. Normally only one judge presides, but for some unexplained reason, two judges were assigned to my case—Rachelle Robles and Linda Burgess.

The initial hearing was scheduled for a year following the filing of the complaint, during the week of April 29, 2024. We attempted mediation in January of 2024 without success. In March 2024, Board staff amended the complaint, dropping the charge of a HIPAA violation; and over time, three more complaints were also dropped. In April 2024, my designated expert, Dr. Richard Urso, became ill. We requested a continuance, and soon after, Dr. Pierre Kory was designated as my expert. The hearing was postponed for six more months and rescheduled for October 2024.

Worn down by the process with legal fees racking up, I decided to let my attorneys go and represent myself pro se. The administrative court system seemed stacked against me, and I concluded that no matter how good my lawyers were, I was going to lose. My attorneys, Steve Mitby and Michael Barnhart, asked me to reconsider, believing they had a good shot at winning, and agreed to represent me pro bono going forward. I accepted their offer.

During the brief period I represented myself, Board attorney Amy Swanholm tried to deceive me into accepting a settlement that would have left a permanent mark on my record. She offered an "agreed order" mandating twelve hours of CME (increased from eight), a public reprimand, and completion of the jurisprudence exam. When I asked if this would stay on my record, she said, "It is a public action, yes. However, after completing the terms, the order would be publicly terminated, and your profile would reflect that it is no longer active." Though she made it sound inconsequential, a quick Google search clarified that an agreed order is a permanent disciplinary action with significant career consequences for physicians. I reported Swanholm to the State Bar of Texas for unethical behavior, but the outcome remains unknown.

This experience with the Board's attorney highlights a broader pattern of inconsistency in how the Texas Medical Board handles disciplinary actions. Of its nineteen members, two have faced discipline from their own Board, and one is under FTC scrutiny. Both disciplined members received remedial plans, which, unlike agreed orders, are nondisciplinary settlements for minor violations with minimal career impact. Dr. Devinder Bhatia, a Houston cardiothoracic surgeon, was sued for assault after allegedly grabbing, hitting, and shoving a nurse in the operating room. The lawsuit settled, and the Board issued him a remedial plan with a $500 fine and twelve hours of continuing education, effectively avoiding discipline. This was not Bhatia's first issue; in 2014, he failed to report on his license renewal that he was under investigation following resignations from two hospitals.

The Texas Medical Board's lenient handling of Dr. Bhatia's case reflects a broader trend of minimal accountability for its own members. Dr. Satish Nayak, another Board member, received a remedial plan for failing to maintain adequate medical records for multiple patients. His penalty was limited to completing eight hours of continuing education on proper recordkeeping, a minor consequence compared to the severe agreed orders imposed on other physicians.

This pattern of leniency extends to the Board's leadership, raising further concerns about its integrity. Dr. Sherif Zaafran, the Board's president, serves as vice chairman of U.S. Anesthesia Partners' (USAP) clinical governance board for Texas's Gulf Coast region and as USAP's national legislative liaison. The FTC is currently suing USAP, Texas's largest anesthesia firm, for alleged price gouging and monopolistic practices. Despite an appeal to the Fifth Circuit, the lawsuit against USAP remains active,[1] casting a shadow over Zaafran's leadership.

The Texas Medical Board's questionable oversight extends to its handling of expert witnesses. In July 2024, Dr. Irvin Zeitler, former Texas Medical Board president and the Board's expert, became too ill to testify. For his preparation, Dr. Zeitler charged the TMB a flat fee of $15,422. Through open records requests, I discovered he significantly inflated his fees for my case compared to another case that year, where he charged the TMB a flat fee of $4,775. In 2023, the average compensation for TMB expert witnesses was $4,096.94, revealing that Dr. Zeitler's fee for my case was substantially higher.

After Dr. Zeitler withdrew from the case, the ALJs granted a second continuance, delaying the hearing by an additional seven months until May 2025. Open records requests show the Board paid 450 experts nearly $1.5 million in fees in 2023, indicating a robust pool of available and well-paid experts. Despite this, the Board claimed it needed over six months to secure a replacement for this case.

On October 22, 2024, the Board designated Dr. Alex Gilman, DO, to take Dr. Zeitler's place. Less than three months later, Dr. Gilman suddenly withdrew. Like Dr. Zeitler, he charged the Board $15,422 in fees without ever testifying. Board staff wrote:

> Expert communicated to Board Staff that he has chosen to withdraw from his contract to offer testimony on behalf of Board Staff in this matter. He has withdrawn due to public developments regarding individuals connected to this contested case hearing. He is understandably uncomfortable with becoming the target of individuals who seek to intimidate and influence this matter through ancillary pressure on individuals, such as himself, who would offer sworn testimony on behalf of Board Staff.

A month later, on November 27, 2024, the Board filed a confidential Motion for Summary Judgement. We requested oral arguments, which the judges denied.

During this time, I was filing numerous open records requests in preparation for a potential lawsuit against both the FSMB and TMB. In response, on January 7, 2025, Board staff filed a Motion to Protect, writing, "Beginning around April 25, 2024, Respondent began submitting requests for information to the Texas Medical Board's Open Records staff. To date, Respondent has made 117 requests for information under the Public Information Act. On December 31, 2024, alone, Respondent submitted 24 requests for information to TMB Open Records."

The judges never ruled on this, and I continued my requests. To thwart me, the Board changed their fee schedule, demanding I pay in advance before performing a preliminary search on my requests, claiming "the Board has a yearly limit on time that personnel of the governmental body are required to spend producing public information without charging for subsequent requests." I successfully appealed this to Attorney General Ken Paxton, who reprimanded them, stating I did not have to pay a deposit for ongoing requests.

Following the abrupt departure of Dr. Gilman, the Board designated its medical director, Dr. Robert Bredt, as their new expert witness. Their motion included Dr. Bredt's CV (curriculum vitae), which I fortuitously read. I was shocked to find he had served as the lab director for Planned Parenthood throughout his twelve-year tenure with the Board. I went public with the information on X, and Rep. Brian Harrison and Rep. Briscoe Cain both wrote letters to the Texas Medical Board calling for his immediate termination. Within twenty-four hours, Dr. Bredt resigned from his position as medical director of the Texas Medical Board and withdrew as an expert in my case.

The Board tried and failed three times to find an expert willing to testify against me, but on March 12, 2025, SOAH granted the Texas Medical Board partial summary judgment, ruling I knowingly sent a nurse to the hospital without having privileges. The hearing scheduled for April 28, 2025, was repurposed to focus on "aggravating and mitigating factors" the judges would consider in determining my penalty. To prevent further public scrutiny, TMB quietly dropped all other complaints, preventing a hearing on those issues. Additionally, TMB filed a motion to limit the hearing's duration and exclude my exhibits and witnesses.

The hearing opened with attorney Amy Swanholm questioning my social media activity. She asked, "You're quite active on social media, aren't you?" and pressed me to estimate my daily posting frequency. She then focused on specific tweets, beginning with my reply to an account named "Knobby Knees," who posted, "Give it to him through family/friends. Have an anonymous person secretly show them how much and when to sneak it to him in the hospital. These are desperate times, and breaking these illegal rules is the only way."

On X, I responded to Knobby Knees, "He's on his stomach on a vent, and with a feeding tube. Would be hard to sneak it in." Amy asked me to explain what I meant by that, to which I replied, "I have never met 'KnobbyKnees,' I don't know who 'KnobbyKnees' is, and I don't remember this comment. I'm just now looking at it for the first time in three and a half years. So it was—I don't know. It doesn't seem very relevant to what happened."

Amy responded, "Would you condone someone who might be engaging in that type of actions with the patient?"

I replied, "No, and I did not tell anybody to sneak anything in."

For over two hours, Amy continued to press me on my social media activity, dissecting posts I made on X years earlier, with the intent to portray me as a physician who encourages lawbreaking. Toward the end of my testimony, she asked what I would do differently. I explained the case with Mr. Jones was a unique situation I had never faced and likely never would again, that I did my best under the stress of a complex legal battle, and if this were to happen again, I would hire my own attorney to better navigate the circumstances. Unsatisfied, she rephrased and repeated the question multiple times. Seven times, I reiterated the only thing I would have done differently is hire my own attorney if such a situation arose again.

She then brought up a brand-new allegation that had never been discussed previously, claiming I was no longer board certified in Otolaryngology. AAO-HNS did state I am board certified but not up-to-date on my CMEs, and I am also board certified, without any CME issues, with the National Board of Physicians and Surgeons (NBPAS). I explained that I had simply failed to upload my CMEs to the AAO-HNS website, but she persisted with this claim in her closing arguments to the judges, citing it as an example of me posing potential harm to the public.

In their summary judgement decision, the administrative law judges held I violated the Medical Practice Act by sending a nurse to administer treatment at Huguley Hospital without having privileges. Their conclusion completely disregarded the fact that the hospital ignored a court order, and in the midst of an active lawsuit, I relied on the advice of the attorney managing the case. TMB originally claimed I did not have a valid physician-patient relationship with Mr. Jones but dropped that complaint. Hence, as Mr. Jones was my patient, I had a legal and ethical obligation to treat him in the manner I believed was in his best interest. By sending a nurse, I was following the Texas Medical Act, not violating it, since ignoring Mr. Jones would have been a dereliction of my duty to my patient.

The judges' decision states I am "subject to discipline because she—without hospital privileges in Huguley Hospital—dispatched her nurse to give the drug to Patient in the Hospital, thereby behaving in a disruptive manner towards hospital personnel that interfered with patient care or was reasonably expected to adversely impact the quality of care rendered to a patient." Nurse Witzel recorded the encounter in the ICU waiting room, showing she behaved responsibly, and there is no evidence that a single patient—or anyone else—was adversely impacted by her presence.

Caught in a difficult situation, I sought to balance my obligation to treat Mr. Jones and the hospital's prerogatives, relying on the counsel of an experienced attorney, Beth Parlato, but Board Staff has sought to turn my good faith effort to treat my patient into a major event, asking the ALJs to find aggravating factors to support more significant discipline by the Texas Medical Board.

According to Board Staff, my "unprofessional behavior" demonstrates increased potential for harm to the public and "diminished rehabilitative potential." My social media usage has weighed heavily in their arguments, claiming "communications indicate disruptive conduct in relation to her practice of medicine and her individual obligations as a licensed physician in Texas.… She repeatedly posted comments on social media describing and referencing individuals 'sneaking' prescription drugs to patients who had not been prescribed those drugs." Board Staff took these statements out of context, failed to acknowledge I never directed anyone to sneak anything in, and provided no evidence linking social media posts generally, much less mine, to any increase of potential harm to the public.

Board Staff also argued this statement I made on social media, "TMB should exonerate me, but won't because they have an agenda," is further grounds for increasing my punishment. When Amy questioned me about this, I responded, "Given how long this process has taken, it has not been expeditious, it's been very expensive. So it doesn't feel like… looking at other cases that the medical board disciplines, the notifications I get of other doctors who are sex offenders and drug addicts, and it's just hard for me to believe that this process has taken so long, has been so expensive, over this matter. So it does feel like there's an agenda."

Amy pressed me to be more specific, to which I responded, "Well, I—as I said, it feels political, because the entire pandemic became political. It wasn't about the patient. It wasn't about saving the life of a patient, sticking up for a patient. It is, you know, it seems, driven by some other agenda."

During cross-examination, my attorney revealed that the hospital filed a complaint against me with the Board before the alleged incident—dispatching Nurse Witzel to administer ivermectin on November 10, 2021—had even occurred, as the hospital's complaint was submitted ten days earlier. Furthermore, Board members were emailing and texting about my case before the initial informal settlement conference. In fact, they filed a complaint against me before I testified on behalf of Mr. Jones at the hearing.

The Board's biased handling of my case, marked by premature complaints and internal discussions, is further contradicted by its public claims. Dr. Sherif Zaafran, the Board's president, wrote to Texas Senator Bob Hall that, "no licensee has faced discipline or excessive scrutiny from the Board for properly prescribing a particular treatment (including Ivermectin, HCQ, and Budesonide), off-label or not, for COVID-19." Board staff and judges echoed this in closing arguments and their decision. Yet, during my deposition, the word "ivermectin" was mentioned eighty-six times, and three of the four complaints I received from the Board specifically cited "ivermectin."

The Board's contradictory stance on ivermectin, as articulated by Dr. Zaafran, aligns with broader pressures from its leadership's affiliations. Dr. Zaafran and TMB Executive Director Stephen Brint Carlton hold leadership roles in the Federation of State Medical Boards (FSMB), which, on July 29, 2021, issued a press release warning that spreading medical misinformation could lead to license revocation. Three months later, on November 1, 2021, I received my first complaint from Texas Huguley Hospital, followed by three more from Houston Methodist Hospital on December 22, 2021, January 19, 2022, and September 7, 2023. The last two complaints, which required informal settlement conference meetings, were dismissed. One stemmed from the mother of a seventeen-year-old boy with a kidney transplant history, whose father requested ivermectin as a precaution for a European trip. As ivermectin is metabolized by the liver, not the kidneys, and the boy was not on conflicting medications, he faced no increased risk.

The pattern of complaints against me, influenced by the Texas Medical Board's leadership ties to the FSMB, culminated in a final grievance in September 2023 from a pharmacist who refused to fill my prescriptions for hydroxychloroquine and ivermectin. She falsely claimed I used abusive language and threatened her during a brief phone call, which was witnessed by a friend while I was on vacation. I simply informed her that I would report her to the Texas Pharmacy Board for refusing to fill valid prescriptions. The patient later told me the pharmacist cited my suspension of privileges at Houston Methodist Hospital as a reason for her refusal. I reported her, prompting a Pharmacy Board investigation, the outcome of which remains unknown.

As evidenced by my experience, when physicians who challenge medical orthodoxy face relentless scrutiny, trust in the systems meant to protect both practitioners and patients is destroyed. I could have succumbed to the demands of the Texas Medical Board long ago but am continuing to fight on principle. The final outcome will determine who has more power in the state of Texas: the hospital or the physician acting on behalf of his or her patient.

CHAPTER 11

Injuries

By the time the FDA granted Emergency Use Authorization of the Pfizer COVID shots on December 11, 2020, I had treated well over a thousand COVID patients, primarily using monoclonal antibodies, and any initial fears I might have had about falling seriously ill from COVID were long gone. I contracted COVID very early during the pandemic, responded quickly to hydroxychloroquine, and since I had natural immunity, didn't see any need to get the vaccine. That being said, the same open mind I had about using ivermectin allowed me to entertain the possibility the COVID shots might be beneficial. After sending out a survey to my patients regarding their intentions on getting it, I was surprised by some of the vehement responses I received. Many instinctually knew the danger and would not even consider it.

Early on, I was dubious about the vaccine's efficacy but assumed it was safe. Though I didn't fully trust drug companies, I still believed our federal health agencies did their job of protecting the public from unethical pharmaceutical company practices. I was naive about the financial conflicts of interest and liability protections surrounding these experimental products, factors that should have been fully revealed—but weren't—to those considering getting them.

In terms of efficacy, the lofty promises made by the pharmaceutical companies and parroted by mainstream media seemed too good to be true and prompted me to scrutinize the studies. I started with Pfizer since it was getting the most publicity. I noticed a fundamental flaw with the design—the test subjects were not uniformly and systematically tested for COVID following administration of vaccine and placebo. Though there were criteria for testing, the physician was the ultimate decision-maker on who needed to be tested. Wrong as it was, at that time we were counting patients who tested positive for COVID as having the disease even if their symptoms were mild or absent, and logically, the vaccine studies should have reflected that real-world practice.

Seeking more information, I listened to a group of doctors discuss the vaccines on a podcast called *This Week in Virology*. Since they did not discuss the study design flaw I was worried about, I emailed them (this was in early January 2021), hoping they would address my concern. Not surprisingly, my email went unanswered. The issue nagged at me though, and whenever anyone asked for my opinion on the shots, I cited the flawed study design as a potential problem and a reason to be cautious.

I saw "breakthrough cases" before injuries, and though I didn't recommend the vaccine to any of my patients, I publicly didn't raise concerns until the summer of 2021. Doing a lot of testing, I quickly realized the shots weren't living up to the "95 percent effective" claim. As I collected the vaccination status and symptoms of patients getting tested, a concerning trend soon became obvious—the vaccinated outnumbered the unvaccinated and were just as sick, if not sicker, than the unvaccinated.

I didn't start hearing about or personally seeing injuries from the COVID shots until the fall of 2021. On November 6, 2021, I watched an online COVID conference where Dr. Robert Malone, one of the inventors of mRNA technology, explained exactly how the shots work.

To help understand, a brief review of cellular protein synthesis and how the COVID shots are designed to work is helpful. Cells in our bodies create proteins, and this process begins in the nucleus through transcription of DNA into mRNA. The mRNA leaves the nucleus and travels to ribosomes within the cytoplasm of the cell. Ribosomes then translate the mRNA to create a protein.

The COVID shots are modified mRNA (each uridine in modified mRNA is replaced with N1-methyl-pseudouridine to make it more stable) that codes for spike protein. This mRNA prompts cells throughout the body to create the most toxic portion of the COVID-19 virus, the spike protein. Previous mRNA vaccines have failed because RNA is easily degraded by enzymes before reaching the site of action, and the negatively charged backbone of RNA makes it difficult to cross cell membranes. To overcome these issues, a shell of lipid nanoparticles (LNPs) is used to protect the mRNA and carry it across the cell membrane. LNPs carry the mRNA to the cytoplasm of lymphocytes and other cells where spike protein is synthesized and displayed to other immune system cells (T and B cells) to trigger the immune response. LNPs allow mRNA to permeate cells and distribute widely throughout the body, even the blood-brain barrier.[1]

The mRNA in these shots was specifically modified to evade destruction from the body's natural defense systems. The experts claimed the product stayed in or near the arm, but thanks to the protective lipid nanoparticle shell, modified mRNA has been found throughout the body, including the brain, adrenal glands, reproductive organs, and breast milk.[2] Additionally, the replacement of uridine with N1-methyl-pseudouridine prevents the modified mRNA from rapid breakdown.[3] No study exists showing the modified mRNA is broken down or leaves the body. Evidence of persistent spike protein from the shots has been found as long as 709 days following inoculation.[4] This suggests that the modified mRNA from the COVID shots is still producing spike protein years after introduction into the body.

The lipid nanoparticles used in Pfizer's shot had never been used in any licensed drug before, and their quality control standards have not been disclosed. LNPs are known to cause inflammation,[5] clotting,[6] and found to be toxic when multiple doses are given.[7] The CDC and FDA have stated that mRNA cannot enter the nucleus and integrate with DNA, but LNPs have been shown in studies to facilitate entry of molecules across the nuclear membrane, potentially leading to integration with cellular DNA.[8]

The shots also contain the stabilizing additives PEG (polyethylene glycol) and polysorbate 80. Both products are considered allergenic and associated with incidents of anaphylaxis after the shots. Studies have shown an unexpectedly high incidence of anaphylaxis after the COVID shots, compared to other vaccines, at a rate of 2.5 to 11.1 reactions per million doses.[9] Documenting an allergy to PEG and/or polysorbate 80 was the only way to claim a medical exemption from these shots during the pandemic.

Dr. Malone's lecture was eye-opening and a turning point for me. Others who spoke that day, including physicians Dr. Pierre Kory and Dr. John Littell, provided important clinical testimonials that further heightened my concerns. I knew none of the doctors who presented at the conference, but their observations matched mine.

Dr. Littell said mandated children vaccinations are a "slap in the face" to parents' rights to determine health care for their children—and to the child's "robust immune system," which will be "usurped by a snippet of mRNA and never have the chance to develop natural immunity, with unknown and potentially deadly consequences."[10]

Dr. Pierre Kory, chief medical officer of the Front Line COVID-19 Critical Care Alliance (FLCCC) said, "The vaccines are so toxic, and it's unbelievable they're going after the kids. The adverse event rates are through the roof. The chief one is myocarditis. The chances of being hospitalized with myocarditis caused by the COVID vaccine is something like four to seven times higher than the chance of being hospitalized with COVID."[11]

Armed with more information about the potential dangers of the shots, I sent an email to my patients warning them about the dangers, particularly in regard to children. The marketing service I used to send out the email, Square, later erased my email (without notice), removing all record of it, but I still have the feedback from my patients, mostly positive. The email was cited in future news articles as one of the reasons Houston Methodist Hospital suspended my privileges.

Mandates at Houston Methodist Hospital started April 1, 2021, at which point only 17 percent of Americans had received the COVID shots.[12] The bulk of the country did not get the COVID shots until Biden issued a mandate for all large businesses on September 9, 2021.[13] The following winter, patients started coming in to see me with a constellation of unusual but similar symptoms whose onset occurred shortly after receiving the shots. As the number of patients coming in increased and I started seeing a pattern, I began to speak out publicly. In late February 2022, I tweeted, "8.9% of the patients I saw in the past week were for vaccine injuries."

My first two injured patients were on the milder side—one complained of altered smell immediately after his second Pfizer shot and the other complained of new-onset bilateral tinnitus following his second shot of Moderna—but with time, the injuries I was seeing increased in number and severity. In December, I saw two more injured patients, one with generalized fatigue, dyspnea on exertion, and joint pain, and another patient with POTS. POTS—postural orthostatic tachycardia syndrome—causes blood pressure and heart rate to rise and fall, often dramatically, without any provocation. Symptoms include racing heart and feeling faint when standing. It has become one of the most common injuries I've seen and is very difficult to treat.

Both were previously healthy, middle-aged men whose symptoms started within two weeks of receiving the COVID shot. They had had extensive workups from other physicians with no explanation as to why they were so sick. Their other physicians willfully ignored the relevant history of having had a recent COVID shot and did not report them to VAERS. In fact, at this point, I've seen hundreds of vaccine-injured patients, and not one of them has been reported to VAERS by other providers.

VAERS is the Vaccine Adverse Event Reporting System, a national program managed by the CDC and FDA to monitor the safety of vaccines after they are licensed. Anyone—healthcare providers, patients, or the public—can submit reports of adverse reactions after vaccination to help identify potential safety concerns for further investigation. All vaccine providers were bound by their vaccine provider agreement and the False Claims Act to report adverse events arising from the COVID shot to VAERS.

A study from Harvard analyzed 1.4 million vaccine doses given to 376,452 patients from June 2006 to October 2009, identifying 35,570 possible adverse reactions (2.6 percent of vaccinations). The study estimated that fewer than 1 percent of vaccine adverse events are reported to VAERS due to the system's passive nature and barriers like incomplete recognition and administrative challenges.[14]

As an ENT, I don't administer vaccines and was not even aware of this system prior to the pandemic, but the findings of this Harvard study are consistent with what I have been seeing in my office since the COVID shots entered the market. Patients with suspected or obvious injuries are not being reported by other providers. VAERS was meant for the situation at hand—a vaccine rushed to the market using brand-new technology—but most people didn't even know about it. Surgeons General Jerome Adams and Vivek Murthy, as holders of the official microphone for our public health system, could have used their positions to educate physicians and the general public about VAERS, but they never did.

Moreover, those who did what they were obligated to do and reported possible injuries to VAERS risked professional consequences. In October 2021, physician's assistant Deborah Conrad was fired and publicly escorted out of Rochester Regional Health (employed by United Memorial Medical Center) for reporting COVID vaccine adverse events to VAERS. She writes:

> When I noticed several adverse events, including death, post-vaccination, I began writing and submitting patient reports to VAERS in my spare time. I was asked several times to 'dial it back' and to only create reports for my own patients, not those whom other providers treated. Rochester Regional Health asked me to 'tow the company line', which was to support the vaccine and reduce vaccine hesitancy, despite their legal obligation to report vaccine injuries.[15]

From 2022 onward, patients with a variety of symptoms, including intractable chest pain, brain fog, tremors, rashes, blood clots, and new-onset neuropathy, have trickled into my office seeking help. In the two years following the rollout of the COVID shots, approximately 7 percent of my new patients came to see me for injuries. Even now, not a day goes by where I don't see someone who was injured or hear from a patient about a close friend or relative who was. Last week (May 2025), I saw four injured patients in one day. Today, working only a half-day, I saw two.

As an ENT, I'm used to fixing people quickly. The most rewarding aspect of my job is seeing people significantly improve with a short course of medication or a surgical procedure, and it's one of the reasons I chose a surgical specialty and not primary care. COVID was new but predictable, and because of the large number of patients coming in day after day, I was able to master it in a short period of time. Treating COVID patients aligned with the practice approach I was accustomed to, as patients responded very well in a short amount of time to a relatively short course of treatment using a few medications.

COVID vaccine injuries, on the other hand, have been far more difficult to manage, as patients do not respond to treatment as predictably and quickly as the disease itself. Much of the approach is trial and error, but I typically start with ivermectin as it binds spike protein and has anti-inflammatory properties. The Independent Medical Alliance (formerly FLCCC) has a protocol which I follow,[16] but patients are still very slow to recover.

The number of people injured from the COVID shots is far greater than what our public health system is willing to recognize. Apart from the problem of underreporting to VAERS, the majority of doctors won't even entertain the possibility that these patients' symptoms could be related to the vaccine. Patients go through an extensive workup, only to result in normal labs and imaging studies, prompting the physicians to conclude they are suffering from a psychiatric condition. I've seen numerous people clearly injured from the shots who were cast aside by other physicians and given prescription antidepressants, anxiety medications, and sleeping pills.

Another fundamental problem is the absence of an ICD-10 code for adverse events from the COVID shots (ICD-10 refers to the 10th edition of the International Classification of Diseases, a medical coding system designed by the World Health Organization to categorize health conditions). Every known disease is assigned a specific ICD-10 code used by Medicare and insurance companies for billing and tracking; without an ICD-10 code, the disease basically doesn't exist and cannot be tracked.

We live in an unfortunate era where a clinician's assessment is not enough for a diagnosis. Doctors today won't treat without a test to confirm the diagnosis, and routine tests are typically not helpful in diagnosing those injured by the COVID shot. The one test I've found useful, which most other doctors don't order, is Labcorp's spike protein antibody test. The spike protein is the pathogenic portion of the virus, and I have found that levels correlate with the level of symptoms. Though antibodies do not directly measure spike protein in the body, higher levels suggest higher levels of spike protein. Specialized labs are able to measure actual spike protein levels, but this test is not available to the general public.

Historically, we've used antibody levels to determine immunity status from certain infections. But because this virus mutates so quickly, spike protein antibody levels have not correlated well with protection from infection. In other infections, this is not the case. Healthcare professionals working in a hospital often have to prove immunity to hepatitis B, for example, by showing antibody titers. Antibody titers typically wane over time, and if low, a booster might be required.

Unlike other vaccines, in patients who have had the COVID shots, antibody levels do not seem to wane over time and remain very high years later. Though the test does not distinguish between antibodies from natural infection versus antibodies formed from the shot, at this point, most people have been infected and have some degree of natural antibody production.

In a recent analysis of 129 patients I tested, the average antibody level was 1,323 in forty-six unvaccinated patients and 13,427 in eighty-three vaccinated patients. Though results could be confounded by the presence of recent infection, none of these patients have had a COVID shot in the last three years. The only lab that I know of that provides this test is Labcorp, and the upper limit of testing is twenty-five thousand. I have many patients whose results are greater than twenty-five thousand, meaning the levels were beyond the upper limit of their test capabilities. Hence, the average antibody level of 13,427 is actually an underestimation and could be much higher. The test is currently available without a doctor's order for approximately $69. Quest has a similar test but does not go beyond 2,500, so I don't recommend it.

The high antibody levels suggest persistent spike protein in the body, mostly likely from continued production by the cells. The modified mRNA containing pseudouridine does not break down easily and is likely continuing to prompt cells to make spike protein. I have seen high antibody levels in the unvaccinated after an infection. High levels could also be explained by shedding or from unknown vaccination (many suspect hospitals vaccinated patients without their consent). By and large, though, the vast majority of unvaccinated patients have spike protein antibody levels far below those of the vaccinated.

Vaccine injuries are more challenging to treat than any other disease I've encountered in my career, but of all the things I've tried, I've seen the most improvement using ivermectin. With prolonged use, antibody levels gradually go down, but more importantly, patients feel better. I've had several patients with severe rashes that did not respond to antihistamines or steroids respond very well to ivermectin. That being said, we need more studies to help the injured, particularly those with neurological injuries which are more difficult to treat. We have band aids but need a cure, and we must figure out how to detect and destroy the modified mRNA in the cells. A good resource for supplements and other measures you can try to heal from spike protein is Independent Medical Association's website, www.imahealth.org.

Another great source for people injured from the COVID shots is React19, an organization started by Brianne Dressen and Dr. Joel Wallskog, who both suffered severe debilitating injuries from COVID shots. In addition to educational resources for the injured, React19 has distributed over $1.2 million to help 165 vaccine-injured people. The government, on the other hand, through the CICP (Countermeasures Injury Compensation Program), has denied 98 percent of applications from injured patients. As of this writing, only thirty-nine people have received compensation. If you take out two outliers (one was awarded $370,000 and another received over $2 million), the remaining thirty-seven have been awarded an average of only $4,648.99 each.[17]

CHAPTER 12

Censorship

Five years ago, the government decided they knew better than your doctor. Bureaucrats like Anthony Fauci and Rochelle Walensky—with no clinical experience treating COVID patients—collectively decided your doctor, no matter how many years in practice, papers published, or lives saved, was not competent. These government doctors invaded our exam rooms, hijacked your right to bodily autonomy and informed consent, and—without a vote—declared themselves the experts. They were the science, and they were in charge.

The power grab was remarkable given their lack of clinical experience. Despite their degrees, none of them practice medicine. None of them examined COVID patients, took histories, or wrote prescriptions. None of them cared for a single COVID patient. But because they had the full support of Big Pharma, the government, and most importantly the media, they became the scientific authority on a novel disease they had zero firsthand experience in treating. They dictated who would get treated and how—all from the safety of their homes, over Zoom calls, never risking their own lives to care for a single COVID patient.

On July 15, 2021, Surgeon General Vivek Murthy issued an official advisory letter concerning the dangers of misinformation, asking social media companies to "consistently take action against misinformation super-spreaders."[1] Two weeks later, the FSMB, a private organization with self-declared oversight over all state medical boards, issued a policy statement warning that doctors who spread medical misinformation could lose their medical license.[2] In the following months, a flurry of doctors across the country, including myself, received complaints from their respective boards. As "misinformation" lacks codification in state statutes, boards found other avenues to pursue, often using "unprofessional conduct" as a way to take action against ivermectin prescriptions.

Misinformation is defined as false or inaccurate information, but during the pandemic, it morphed into meaning anything that countered the government's narrative. As evidenced by the actions taken against me and numerous other healthcare professionals who disagreed with the CDC and FDA, scientific debate was stifled when it was needed most. This suppression of dissenting voices forced many physicians, already cautious about public engagement, to remain silent. As a rule, physicians typically maintain a low public profile, hesitant to advertise or engage on social media due to ethical concerns. In contrast, pharmaceutical companies, hospitals, and insurers face no such restrictions, and during the pandemic, they dominated public discourse. Houston Methodist's billboards line every major highway near my office, and with widespread radio and TV ads, their brand is inescapable.

Launching my practice, I cautiously engaged on social media, careful to be truthful and avoid sensationalism. I periodically posted my COVID test results online but with zero commentary. As I became more connected with like-minded physicians online, and as my patient experiences started veering away from what the government and media were telling everyone, I became more outspoken. I was, and still am, careful to post facts I've personally observed or that are backed by reputable sources.

In the summer of 2021, I asked Mas Takashima with Houston Methodist Hospital if he was seeing the same trend of "breakthrough" cases I was seeing. I only started sharing the information on social media after he dismissed my concerns. On August 1, I tweeted, "Of the 32 positives we saw in July, half were in fully vaccinated people. 3 people had had previous COVID-19, and 1 of those had also been vaccinated." My posts back then were far more cautious than they are today, stating things such as "Ivermectin works" and "Vaccine mandates are wrong." It felt like whispering in a storm though, as few people liked or commented on what I was saying.

Lacking local support, I turned to Twitter to connect with other physicians treating COVID patients. Dr. Mollie James, a St. Louis-based general surgeon and critical care physician, became an ally. Her work in New York's COVID ICUs led her to question hospital protocols. Barred from using treatments like ivermectin, she developed home care protocols, saving lives, including her brother's, and later founded The James Clinic to focus on preventive care and vaccine injury treatment. Other allies, like Dr. Lynn Fynn and Dr. Kat Lindley, shared similar experiences, adding to my growing network of dissenting physicians.

Outspoken physicians and advocates quickly formed a tight-knit community on X, including nonphysicians using pseudonyms like TexasLindsay (now Lindsay Penney), The Vigilant Fox, UngaTheGreat, Chief Nerd, and Gain of Fauci. Over time, these allies evolved into credible independent media voices with significant followings. My own account remained modest until 2021, when Houston Methodist's critical tweets and media alerts unexpectedly amplified my visibility. Through notoriety, their efforts inadvertently elevated my message. However, as my voice and others like mine gained traction, powerful forces moved to silence us, framing our dissent as dangerous misinformation and leveraging vast resources to control the narrative.

The COVID-19 Community Corps was not a simple public awareness initiative—it was an orchestrated attack against free speech. Billions of dollars were distributed to battalions of media influencers incentivized and rewarded with our tax dollars to censor, silence, and attack anyone with dissenting opinions. Consequently, the voices of frontline nurses, physician assistants, and physicians like myself who were seeing, treating, researching, and collaborating—doing everything we could to help—were not only buried, but many of us had to fight to keep our licenses. This attack included innocent civilians, patients, and concerned citizens, many of whom were injured by the protocols and shots they were coerced into taking. Journalists who tried to give us a voice were punished—fired, demonetized, and deplatformed. We were kicked off Twitter (now X), Facebook, Instagram, TikTok, YouTube, and LinkedIn, and to this day, I still can't give an interview that airs on YouTube without risk of the journalist getting deplatformed. In an interview I recently did with Jimmy Dore (May 2025), my comments on the vaccine were bleeped out, a precaution Jimmy took to prevent YouTube from demonetizing his account. In August 2025, I opened another TikTok account, curious to see if the company had loosened its censorship policies. My account lasted less than a month.

Our country has not always enjoyed the right to free speech. In colonial America, dissenters faced imprisonment or worse for challenging authorities. Under colonial religious code, attending the Anglican church—referred to as the established "state" church—was mandated. Anyone practicing a different form of Christianity was called a "dissenter," and many were arrested, beaten, exiled, and even hung for daring to speak out. It took about a hundred years until the first law was proposed to protect religious freedom and free speech in America. In 1786, Thomas Jefferson's Virginia Statute for Religious Freedom became the driving force behind the First Amendment.

Two hundred thirty-four years later, the lessons from the colonial era seem far remote. But a major health crisis set in the digital age served as a critical new test of free speech rights. The cornerstone of our democracy, free speech safeguards the majority from dominating the minority, allows divergent viewpoints to be heard, and prevents secretive government control over information. Protection of free speech is most crucial during times of uncertainty.

Social media offers an unprecedented platform for open debate, giving every individual a megaphone and the right to be heard. But the right to free speech is not limited to individuals. The First Amendment also protects the speech of private social media companies, bestowing upon them the right to ban any content they want. At the same time, they are protected by law from any content that might cause harm. No major lawsuits against social media companies for censorship have succeeded in US courts, primarily due to legal protections under Section 230 of the Communications Decency Act. Section 230 grants platforms immunity from liability for user-generated content and allows them to moderate content in "good faith" without being sued for censorship.

Unable to directly censor Americans due to legal constraints, the government collaborated with social media platforms to moderate content. On March 24, 2021, the Center for Countering Digital Hate (CCDH) released its "Disinformation Dozen" report, identifying top social media accounts, including Robert F. Kennedy Jr., as sources of alleged vaccine misinformation. This report spurred twelve Democratic state attorneys general to urge Twitter and Facebook CEOs to remove these accounts. While CCDH denied receiving US government funding, it openly engaged with government officials like Minnesota Senator Amy Klobuchar to promote censorship strategies. On April 19, 2021, Senator Klobuchar sent a letter to Twitter CEO Jack Dorsey and Facebook CEO Mark Zuckerberg highlighting CCDH's Disinformation Dozen report.[3] Months later, in July 2021, Senator Klobuchar filed the "Health Misinformation Act" that would suspend legal protection of social media companies when they boost "anti-vax" misinformation.[4]

In October 2021, the CEO of CCDH, a British citizen named Imran Ahmed, presented a webinar to the FSMB titled, "Stopping the Spread: Disinformation and Its Impact on Physicians and Patients." Shortly thereafter, on December 13, 2021, Shannon Glueck, PharmD and FDA branch chief at the FDA, sent a letter to the head of FSMB warning about the supposed dangers of ivermectin, stating, "However, the FDA has neither authorized nor approved any ivermectin drug product for use in preventing or treating COVID-19.... Using ivermectin products in preventing or treating COVID-19 may pose risks to patient health or lead to delays in getting effective treatment of COVID-19. Drug products that claim to treat or prevent COVID-19 but are not proven safe and effective for those purposes can place consumers at risk of serious harm."[5]

These efforts to control online discourse intensified as the pandemic's third surge hit, amplifying tensions between official narratives and dissenting voices like mine. By summer 2021, our country was in the midst of the pandemic's third and largest surge. Six months after vaccines became available, only 65 percent of Americans were vaccinated, falling short of the 85 percent target considered necessary to achieve herd immunity. The vaccine was the Hail Mary guaranteed to save us from disease and death, but as cases exploded in the face of this promise, a vocal minority took to social media to sound the alarm. Once I had firm firsthand confirmation, I joined them with gusto.

Our small but mighty army caught the attention of the pandemic overlords. In mid-July, the White House publicly admitted it was working with social media companies to identify "misinformation." Press Secretary Jen Psaki announced, "We are regularly making sure social media platforms are aware of the latest narratives dangerous to public health that we and many other Americans are seeing across all of social and traditional media. And we work to engage with them to better understand the enforcement of social media platform policies."[6] On the same day, Surgeon General Vivek Murthy declared: "We are saying we expect more from our technology companies. We are asking them to operate with greater transparency and accountability.... We are asking them to monitor misinformation more closely. We are asking them to consistently take action against misinformation super spreaders on their platforms."[7]

In the six months following the White House's call to arms, a wave of dissident accounts was suspended across Facebook, Instagram, Twitter, and TikTok. From January 2020 to September 2022, Twitter suspended more than eleven thousand accounts over violations of its COVID misinformation policy, and Meta boasted of removing over sixteen million posts on Facebook and Instagram.[8]

After repeated warnings and temporary suspensions, my Twitter account was "permanently suspended" on July 28, 2022. My final display of dissidence was, "Lawyer up @twitter and @cdc. @america1stlegal obtains emails between CDC director of digital media Carol Crawford and @twitter execs on how to suppress free speech. Examples in thread."[9] The tweet went viral, with twenty-two thousand likes, and that was the last utterance I was allowed from my Twitter account for the ensuing five months. Desperate to keep speaking out, I tried creating alternate accounts with new emails and a VPN, but Twitter kept shutting me down. I posted on Instagram, Truth Social, and Gettr, but nothing matched Twitter's reach. I was forced to spend the next five months in maddening silence.

When the hammer fell, I was in Ireland with fellow medical freedom warriors Mollie James, Kat Lindley, Lynn Fynn, and Lindsey Penney for a Global COVID-19 Summit conference, a gathering of doctors challenging pandemic policies. Post-conference, we staged a protest at Twitter's Dublin headquarters. With righteous indignation, we positioned ourselves outside the office windows of people we thought worked at Twitter, waving neon yellow signs with blue birds and bold messages while throwing fist pumps and glares—only to realize the people we were heckling worked at a different company, and our targets were out of reach.

This exercise in futility did not discourage us for long. Months later, the richest man in America began plotting our escape from the digital dungeon we dubbed "Twitmo." Rumors of Elon Musk buying Twitter kicked off in January 2022, but months of back-and-forth uncertainty felt like a tease, until he finally sealed the deal eight months later on October 27, 2022. That takeover was the pandemic's game changer, springing our voices free from censorship's grip and handing us back our megaphone.

My Twitter ban dragged on for fifty-nine more days, but it ended with a bang. On Christmas morning 2022, the first thing I saw when I checked my phone was a friend's text with a link to my restored account. Stunned, I responded, "Holy shit!" The news brought mixed emotions. Thrilled as I was to have my account back, I knew the memory of that Christmas and all going forward would forever be tangled with Twitter's ban. Now, looking back, I consider the timing as a divine nod, and it brings a smile to my face.

With my voice back, I didn't waste time—I pushed to help my friends. After a quick victory lap, I tweeted at Elon to free my banned comrades, and to my surprise, he delivered. Within twenty-four hours, all twelve accounts I championed were restored: Dr. Mollie James, Dr. Kat Lindley, Dr. Lynn Fynn, Dr. Brian Tyson, Dr. George Fareed, Dr. Craig Wax, Dr. Stella Immanuel, Dr. Ben Marble, Dr. Simon Goddek, Texas Lindsay, and Vigilant Fox. It was a spectacular win after months of suppression.

CHAPTER 13

Suing the FDA

As a private practitioner, I never wasted much time thinking about the FDA, but on March 5, 2021, the FDA invaded my exam room. They fired no shots, but their actions caused many casualties. I fought back, and after a series of attacks and a long occupation, the FDA finally retreated. Reconstruction is ongoing, but FDA overreach into my office—and every doctor's office in America—was halted.

When the Pfizer mRNA shot rolled out in late 2020, the FDA didn't just approve it, they started a campaign to wedge themselves between me and my patients. Every time I prescribed ivermectin, a safe, FDA-approved drug, I felt their overreach like a weight on my pen. They politicized medicine, turning the sacred doctor-patient bond into a battleground, not just in my Texas practice, but across the country.

In my practice, I treated over six thousand COVID patients, saving every one I caught early with a regimen that included ivermectin—a drug the FDA approved for human use in 1987. Whether or not you believe ivermectin is effective for COVID, the point is this: The FDA has no business dictating what doctors prescribe or how doctors care for their patients. Yet they did, with a vengeance, threatening my license and the livelihoods of countless doctors nationwide.

The FDA's job is to approve drugs and their labels, not to play doctor. It's a gatekeeper, not a healer, with no skin in the game for patient outcomes. Yet it weaponized its authority, plastering its website with warnings like, "Why You Should Not Use Ivermectin to Treat or Prevent COVID-19," and FAQs bluntly stating, "No, don't take it." Nowhere did they mention their lack of legal power to dictate prescriptions or block off-label use, leaving patients and doctors in the dark.

On August 21, 2021, as COVID surged, the FDA fired its most infamous shot: a tweet showing a health care worker nuzzling a horse, captioned, "You are not a horse. You are not a cow. Seriously, y'all. Stop it." The media ran with it, branding ivermectin as horse dewormer. That tweet, seen by millions in days, became the FDA's viral middle finger to doctors like me, igniting a firestorm that nearly cost me my license.

My evidence-based stance on ivermectin put a target on my back. The FDA's campaign didn't just threaten my license—it jeopardized my livelihood and my ability to help patients. Pharmacies refused to fill ivermectin prescriptions, insurance companies balked at covering it, and patients, bombarded by "horse dewormer" headlines, begged for reassurance. I told them it is one of the safest drugs I've ever prescribed, but the damage was done.

I wasn't alone. Doctors across the country faced the same gauntlet, and two doctors battling the same FDA roadblocks helped me fight back. Alongside Dr. Robert Apter and Dr. Paul Marik, and represented by Jared Kelson with Boyden Gray, I sued the agency on June 2, 2022. We faced setbacks, but we dug in, fueled by the oath we took—do no harm. The FDA's meddling had broken that vow, forcing us to fight not just for our patients, but for every doctor's right to practice free of bureaucratic chains. On April 6, 2024, after nearly two years and a blistering Fifth Circuit ruling, the FDA backed down, deleting its "You are not a horse" tweet and scrubbing its anti-ivermectin posts.

The war left scars—board complaints still haunt me, and other physicians and patients still have difficulty accessing ivermectin—but we carved out a small shield for future patients against FDA overreach. A full victory would entail correcting the misinformation surrounding ivermectin and exonerating physicians who were unfairly persecuted for prescribing and speaking out about it.

The current FDA has the power not only to educate the public and physicians about the safety and efficacy of ivermectin but also to make it over-the-counter. I've performed two polls on X asking the public where they access their ivermectin, and in both, over 50 percent replied they get it from a feed store, with the second most common response being from another country. The FDA's silence on this matter is leading Americans to take animal medication and potentially putting people in harm's way.

Fourteen states recently proposed legislation to make ivermectin over-the-counter, and as of August 2025, five states—Tennessee, Idaho, Louisiana, Texas, and Arkansas—successfully passed that legislation. Attempts failed in South Carolina, Montana, Kentucky, Maine, West Virginia, Alabama, Oklahoma, Missouri, and Minnesota.

CHAPTER 14

Americans for Health Freedom

COVID directly impacted every single voter in this country, yet the vast majority of people in office and running for office don't wish to talk about it. During the last presidential election, both Trump and Biden tiptoed around the subject, ignoring the largest public health crisis of our lifetime, despite an ongoing and robust dialogue on social media from the voters. This deafening silence from our politicians suggests the hidden hand of Big Pharma holds far more power than the people.

Early in the pandemic, I shied away from politics, worried it would weaken my argument. At the press conference I held following my suspension from Houston Methodist Hospital, I adamantly stated politics has no place in medicine. I believe that was the right call at the time, and I still believe we should separate medicine from politics. But now, with health authorities ignoring irrefutable data concerning the dangers of the COVID shots, I feel I have no choice but to engage with the political system. The people we elected to represent and protect us need to step in and take action.

In 2023, I stumbled upon a post on X from Michigan State Representative Brad Paquette, who shared his personal ordeal with vaccine-induced myocarditis. I knew, because of his experience and position, his voice could have an impact, so I asked him if he'd be willing to publicly call for the COVID shots to be pulled off the market. He wholeheartedly responded, "Yes!" and his response gave me the courage to ask other politicians the same question. To my surprise, many shared similar concerns, leading to a rapidly growing coalition. In just three months, our list of candidates and elected officials calling for the COVID shots to be pulled off the market surged to 255 members, underscoring a widespread and urgent call for action against the backdrop of Big Pharma's influence on our electoral system.

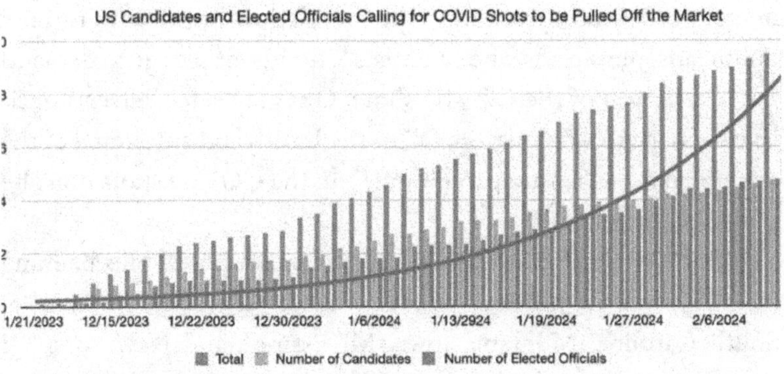

People have argued no one should cast a vote based on a single issue. But in my opinion, a candidate's position on the COVID shots is a strong litmus test. Signing our pledge is politically risky and a sign of strength and integrity. Though many politicians likely got the first set of vaccines, very few continue to follow CDC recommendations and get an annual booster, and very few are willing to take a risk and inject their children or grandchildren with this shot. Yet the vast majority remain silent. If the vaccines aren't safe enough for them or their children, how are they safe enough for their constituents? The hypocrisy is stunning.

Our pledge expanded from simply stating the shots should be pulled off the market to also refusing to take donations from Big Pharma. By having the courage to put their name on this list, these candidates and elected officials are rejecting major funding that most politicians rely on to hold office. We have helped many on our list get elected by boosting them on social media, particularly in Texas, and our goal is to continue to give free publicity to politicians who are willing to take a difficult position.

Toward this effort, I, alongside Dr. Kat Lindley, Dr. Mollie James, Dr. Molly Rutherford, and Brian Roberts, founded Americans for Health Freedom. This 501(c)(4) initiative is dedicated to educating the public regarding the harms of these shots and matters of medical freedom. Our foundational project is to rally politicians, physicians, and scientists around this pledge to demand the withdrawal of the COVID shots. Our goal is to deliver a decisive message to Washington, DC—the health and autonomy of the American populace are paramount, and the COVID shots must be pulled off the market.

This last legislative session, nine states proposed bills banning mRNA shots in humans—Texas, Idaho, Kentucky, Minnesota, South Carolina, Montana, Iowa, Mississippi, and New York. Of these, Montana came the closest, managing to get the bill out of committee, but despite a Republican majority, the bill was voted down in the House, thirty-four to sixty-six. Twenty-four Republicans voted against it. As of this writing, only Michigan, authored by State Representative Brad Paquette, has an active bill banning mRNA in humans.

Americans for Health Freedom is a grassroots organization. We are not backed by big money, but our list has grown thanks to word of mouth on social media. Aside from a few Independents, the politicians who have signed are Republicans, but we are not interested in party politics and welcome Democrats to join our cause. We have politicians with varying levels of power, from school board members and precinct chairs to members of Congress. Of the 535 members of Congress, only three have had the moral courage to sign our pledge—Rep. Thomas Massie (R-KY), Rep. Marjorie Taylor Greene (R-GA), and Sen. Ron Johnson (R-WI)—and sadly, our biggest hope, Secretary of Health and Human Services (HHS), Robert F. Kennedy Jr., never signed. But our list continues to grow, and as of August 2025, we have 256 elected officials, twelve candidates, one surgeon general, one state Republican party, one state congressional district, seventeen Republican Party county committees, and seven physician organizations all pledging to call for the COVID shots to be pulled off the market.

If you would like to help, please share the pledge at www.AmericansforHealthFreedom.org and urge your representatives to sign.

CHAPTER 15

MAHA

The Pfizer-BioNTech and Moderna COVID shots were authorized in November 2021 for ages five to eleven and in June 2022 for ages six months and older, and then they were added to the pediatric immunization schedule on February 9, 2023. The recommendation for all babies to get three COVID shots by the age of nine months remained until May 27, 2025, and 13 percent of American children, amounting to 9.5 million total, received the 2024–2025 version.

When Robert F. Kennedy Jr. was sworn in as Secretary of HHS, he promised to end the chronic disease epidemic in children, and based on his statements made during the pandemic, we assumed that included mRNA. Those of us who have been fighting the injustices of the past five years hoped for immediate action, anticipating he would remove the COVID shots from the market or, at a minimum, discontinue the recommendation to give them to children and pregnant women. Frustrations are growing as his first months in power have gone by without addressing the COVID shots. His policy strategy outlined in a seventy-six-page MAHA (Make America Healthy Again) report on May 22, 2025, did not even mention mRNA, instead focusing on ultra-processed foods, environmental toxins, and over-medicalization of children.

The public's response to his silence has been mixed. One camp of his supporters has chosen to fiercely defend him, assuring the rest of us we should trust the plan, while others criticize his unwillingness to talk about the issue we counted on him to address. Medical freedom doctors and activists have become divided, with many of the ones who know Kennedy on a personal level choosing to defend his inaction. Some doctors, like Robert Malone, have been critical of medical freedom activists like myself who continue to push Kennedy to pull the shots off the market, comparing our persistent outcries to "tantrums." Malone's loyalty was recently rewarded with an appointment to the CDC's Advisory Committee on Immunization Practices (ACIP).

After an enormous amount of public pressure, on May 27, 2025, the CDC finally modified the pediatric vaccine schedule to change COVID shots for children from "recommended" to "shared decision making." Practically speaking, this represents a political compromise more than anything else. Pediatricians can and likely still will advise parents to give their children these shots, and they might use these new guidelines to scare parents into vaccinating children with mild comorbidities guised as COVID risk factors. Further, despite an announcement from Kennedy on X, the general public seems unaware of the change. Today, as I was picking up a prescription for my father at Walgreens, I witnessed a mother bringing her healthy-appearing teenage son into Walgreens to get a COVID booster.

Until recently, these shots were still under EUA status for children under twelve, but they are still protected from liability under the Public Readiness and Emergency Preparedness (PREP) Act.

On May 20, 2025, Drs. Marty Makary and Vinay Prasad published the article "An Evidence-Based Approach to COVID-19 Vaccination" in the *New England Journal of Medicine,* concluding that vaccine companies can still obtain annual licensing with minimal data (only showing an antibody response) for adults older than sixty-five and everyone else (including children) with a single comorbidity. For "healthy" children and adults under sixty-five, the companies will be required to conduct randomized controlled trials to obtain further licensing.[1]

Meanwhile, the COVID virus has evolved into the equivalent of a cold, and like other colds, evolves rapidly to escape immune detection. Chasing strains with new shots simply pressures the virus to continue to evolve and persist. Measuring outcomes from these "vaccines" will be difficult, given the growing rarity of infections and unlikelihood of poor outcomes with infection.

Myocarditis in young males is the only serious adverse event the CDC is willing to admit could occur after the COVID shots. Among males aged twelve to seventeen, CDC reports approximately twenty-two to thirty-six out of every one hundred thousand experienced myocarditis within twenty-one days after receiving a second vaccine dose.[2] A study examining the Vaccine Adverse Event Reporting System (VAERS) found that young males ages fifteen to seventeen had the highest incidence, with 105.9 cases per million doses administered, and the second dose carried the highest risk compared to the first.[3] Another study from Israel estimated the risk at 10.69 per one hundred thousand among adolescents and young adult males who received the mRNA COVID-19 vaccine.[4]

The telltale sign of myocarditis is chest pain, and even with that symptom, myocarditis is difficult to diagnose. The only definitive way is to do a cardiac biopsy, and the next best option is a cardiac MRI, a test which is expensive and not easily available. EKG and blood tests can help but are nonspecific. Most doctors do not entertain the possibility of myocarditis if the patient does not complain of chest pain.

Myocarditis is a significant cause of sudden cardiac death in young adults, with estimates suggesting that up to 20 percent of sudden deaths in this age group may be related to myocarditis.[5] While many people recover, myocarditis can lead to permanent damage to the heart muscle, increasing the risk of complications such as arrhythmias and heart failure. Prior to 2021, the average number of cardiac arrests per year among professional athletes was twenty-nine. This increased ten-fold to 283 per year in 2021.[6]

The data is hard to find, but following the initial rollout, an estimated three hundred twenty-five thousand American children under four received the shots, and presumably hundreds of thousands more have received them since then. The change in recommendations might be used as a marketing tool to increase uptake, given there are an estimated thirty million children with one of the conditions listed as increasing the risk of severe COVID.

Of grave concern is the uncertainty over the number of children who could develop undetected myocarditis following the shots. Babies can't tell you they have chest pain, so the odds a physician will work up a young child for myocarditis following the shots are exceedingly low. Even myocarditis that does not cause initial heart failure can leave a permanent scar on the heart, imparting a lifelong increased risk of sudden death with extreme exertion.

HHS officials have repeatedly stated they need more data to take action and pull the shots off the market. But the data is there if they choose to look at it. The biggest hurdle has not been finding the data, it's been trying to convince anyone with authority to acknowledge and act upon it. In addition to prospective studies, we have passive surveillance data through VAERS, post-marketing confidential EUA safety data, reanalysis of Pfizer and Moderna trials, Defense Medical Epidemiology Database (DMED) data, autopsy studies, life insurance and disability data, and case reports all showing the risks of the mRNA shots outweigh the benefits.[7] The uncertainty over the long-term effects on young children causes me the most concern and seems the most obvious reason to pull the product. I fear we will be seeing more and more young athletes dropping dead from undiagnosed subclinical myocarditis.

Overcoming the willful blindness of government bureaucrats seemed an insurmountable feat, but that changed on April 19, 2023, when Robert F. Kennedy Jr. announced his run for presidency. Our hope was bolstered further when he brought Nicole Shanahan on as his running mate. Both have been outspoken critics of how our government handled the pandemic, and Nicole Shanahan has even tweeted that COVID shots should be pulled off the market.

We knew a Kennedy victory for president was a long shot, but we were overjoyed that someone capable of bringing the injustices of the past four years to light was now holding a gigantic microphone. After years of tireless fighting to get the truth out, Kennedy was our best hope. We were finally on the brink of detonating a nuclear bomb on our enemies. Robert F. Kennedy Jr. was that bomb, and we eagerly prepared to drop him on Big Pharma.

But on August 23, 2024, the mission changed, and the bomb's intended target shifted. Kennedy switched course, dropping out of the race, endorsing Trump, and announcing the birth of MAHA. MAHA—Make America Healthy Again—was sold as a way to make Kennedy more palatable to the average American, and in the process, directed the public's attention away from the dangerous mRNA shots and onto our food supply. With the birth of MAHA, Pfizer and Moderna have faded from focus. The real enemy is now Kellogg's, a foe who started poisoning us decades ago and continues to poison us, albeit at a much slower, and more voluntary, pace. Instead of wiping out the creators of mRNA, we're now poised to drop our nuclear bomb on a far less serious threat—cereal manufacturers.

This strategy shift coincided with the meteoric rise of Casey and Calley Means, who parachuted into the medical freedom movement on May 14, 2024, with their bestselling debut book, *Good Energy*. On average, fifteen hundred books on diet and nutrition are published each year, and only a handful achieve sustained bestseller status. *Good Energy* echoes what many nutrition experts have been saying for quite some time, that processed foods are unhealthy, but their commonsense message miraculously became an overnight sensation after being picked up by big media names such as Tucker Carlson and Joe Rogan.

Calley is a Big Pharma turncoat who now wants to take down the food industry and is credited with convincing Kennedy to drop out of the race and endorse Trump. As if nothing significant happened the last four years, neither he nor his sister have had much to say about the mRNA shots. Until last summer, none of us had heard of Calley Means, but with the launch of his bestselling book, Calley's following on X has grown exponentially from nineteen thousand to three hundred thousand in just six months. With the ear of both Kennedy and Trump, Calley managed to secure a position as a special government employee when Trump took office. Casey, despite not holding an active medical license and never completing her residency, has been picked to become our next surgeon general.

Apart from the success of the book, the siblings appear to be well-connected Washington insiders, thanks to their father, Grady Means, who served in the White House as an assistant to Vice President Nelson Rockefeller. To his credit, Grady was speaking out about the food industry before *Good Energy* was published, and in an article published in *The Hill*,[8] even alluded to the absurdity of making children take the COVID shots to attend school.

Grady presumably paved the way for his son Calley to be invited to join the Council on Foreign Relations, an influential American think tank with a global focus. Calley's other position of influence is his experience working as a lobbyist at Mercury Public Affairs, the same firm headed by Susie Wiles before she accepted the position of Trump's chief of staff. Mercury focuses on high-stakes public strategy, including lobbying and government relations, with Pfizer and Gilead Sciences (the developer of Remdesivir) as clients.

Calley's sister, Casey, is an ENT who trained at Stanford and Oregon Health and Science University (OHSU), but she dropped out of residency in her final year. In interviews, she has stated she left months before completing her training out of disillusionment with the medical system. Recent statements from her former residency directors at OHSU refute this, claiming she left due to anxiety and feeling overwhelmed by the workload. Casey landed very well on her feet and now runs a biotech company called Levels, which raised $12 million in seed funding in November 2020 and is backed by one of the largest venture capital firms in Silicon Valley, a16z. While in college, she worked at 23andMe. Though Calley has downplayed their relationship, Casey recently posted a photo of herself and former CEO of 23andMe Anne Wojcicki, calling her a "wonderful friend." 23andMe has been widely criticized for selling its customers' genetic data to GlaxoSmithKline for $300 million[9] and recently filed for bankruptcy.

Upon a friend's recommendation, I bought the Means' book, *Good Energy*, and was excited to see that Casey was a fellow ENT who also went to Stanford. I have always felt our profession is too eager to operate on patients with chronic sinusitis and consider myself conservative in terms of taking people to the operating room for what I consider an inflammatory problem. I reached out to Casey multiple times on X (we follow each other) but was disappointed and a bit surprised that she never responded.

I wondered if I was being ignored because of my views on COVID, so I decided to search her X account for posts concerning the pandemic. To my dismay, I found nothing, meaning she either scrubbed her account or, strangely, as a doctor active on social media, had no views on the most significant public health event of our time.

I performed the same search on her brother Calley's account and found nothing pertaining to the mRNA shots. I went back to their book, wondering if they mentioned it and realized their health-focused bestseller, despite publication on the heels of the pandemic, was devoid of anything related to COVID.

My antennae were up, and I was not alone. I have a handful of trusted confidantes I communicate with daily, and we all shared the same concerns. Who are the Means? How did they become so popular so quickly? Where were they during the pandemic? Beyond our small group, other doctors felt the same as we did and were starting to grumble.

Since Casey never responded to my messages, I began challenging the Means on X. On September 9, 2024, I posted, "I hope Drs. Casey and Calley Means will use their influence to join us in calling for the COVID shots to be pulled off the market." Calley responded to my tweet in the comments with a sophisticated word salad that seemed intended to deflect and messaged me claiming to have talked about vaccines during his interview with Tucker. He said, "There are forces to bring childhood health to the top of the agenda. What a ridiculous assertion that the message of Casey and me is about seed oils. Where is this animosity coming from?" I never mentioned seed oils in my post and responded:

> I didn't assert that. I like your message. What worries me is the timing and intensity. Bobby Kennedy is the biggest threat to BigPharma they've ever had. Could it be BigPharma is

> diverting the conversation to the food industry? Shifting the blame? I also worry that Casey, as a physician, is mute about the shots. It's a sign that she implicitly has no issue with them. Multiple other doctors who have been fighting since the start of the pandemic have concerns about you and Casey. Prove us wrong.

Calley then provided me a with a tweet showing how Casey has questioned the Hepatitis B vaccine for newborns. We went back and forth, but I could not get him to state the COVID shots were harmful or should be pulled off the market. Following the DMs, he suggested we talk. Our initial call did not go well—he accused me of subjecting him to a purity test, and our conversation was heated. He reached out to talk twice more, seemingly in response to more and more people challenging him and Casey on X. I told him all he really had to do to put people at ease is go on record about the COVID shots. He repeatedly assured me he was on my side, but despite multiple conversations, messages, and even a face-to-face exchange on the *Danny Jones* podcast, Calley still will not go on record to call for removal of the mRNA shots from the market.

I told Calley that I understand his activism is different than mine and have no issue with that. But I also know that if he truly cared about the welfare of our children, he would have an opinion on the mRNA shots and state that. My focus is COVID, but I find the practice of giving children hormones and chopping off their genitals in an effort to change their gender abhorrent, so I speak out publicly on other health issues beyond COVID when I authentically feel compelled to do so.

Misdirection is a common war tactic and form of propaganda, a technique used to distract attention away from a topic. Thanks to the efforts of MAHA, all eyes have shifted to dropping the Robert F. Kennedy Jr. nuclear bomb onto the food industry, while our more immediate and severe threat—mRNA manufacturers—strengthen their forces. I, along with many others, can't help but wonder if Big Pharma orchestrated this sudden change in focus and if the Means siblings are being used—knowingly or unknowingly—to drive this change.

We are way beyond the pandemic, but hundreds of mRNA vaccines are in development and a small portion of these are self-amplifying (saRNA.) India, the European Union, and Japan have already licensed saRNA vaccines for COVID, and in the US, the FDA just awarded fast-track designation for the development of a saRNA vaccine for H5N1. Self-amplifying mRNA vaccines include genetic instructions to enable the mRNA to replicate itself within cells, resulting in more and prolonged antigen production.

Approximately 30 percent of the mRNA products in the pipeline are intended to target cancer. On Trump's second day in office, he invited Larry Ellison to speak at the White House, where he outlined his AI Stargate Project, which would include rapid production of personalized mRNA cancer vaccines. The backlash on X was intense, but President Trump showed no signs of caring.

CHAPTER 16

Texas

Of all the controversies during the pandemic, forcing working citizens and students to choose between their right to bodily autonomy and staying employed or in school was the most egregious, and it all started in Houston, Texas. COVID shot mandates were born in Texas, and to this day, students and volunteers working in hospitals are still subjected to this tyranny.

Many of us took health freedom for granted and were unprepared for the COVID-era infringements on our rights. Reclaiming and securing these rights in Texas, a state known for valuing freedom, has proven challenging. This is particularly surprising given the Texas House's strong Republican majority, with eighty-eight Republicans compared to sixty-two Democrats.

The Texas COVID-19 Vaccine Freedom Act, co-authored by forty representatives, passed out of the House Committee on Public Health with a vote of ten yays to one nay (Ann Johnson, elected by the Texas Medical Center, was the only nay), but it never made it to the floor.

Fierce public support, driven by vocal legislators (Rep. Brian Harrison, Sen. Mayes Middleton, Rep. Steve Toth, Sen. Bob Hall, and Rep. Tony Tinderholt) and warriors from Texans for Vaccine Choice and Texans for Medical Freedom, revived the bill. In the last and third special session, Governor Abbott called for a vote on the bill, and exactly two years to the day after Houston Methodist publicly shamed me for opposing vaccine mandates, the Texas medical establishment faced a well-deserved punch in the face.

The blow was not a knockout punch, however. The Texas COVID-19 Vaccine Freedom Act protected only employees from vaccine mandates, excluding coverage of students and volunteers. Rep. Jeff Leach amended the bill to omit students from the legislation and later falsely claimed the amended bill included them. Speaker Dade Phelan blocked Rep. Brian Harrison's attempts to amend the bill to cover all citizens and a subsequent proposal to include medical school students. Rep. Steve Toth was at least able to increase the fine for violations from $10,000 to $50,000.

The Texas COVID-19 Vaccine Freedom Act became law, and though it's a big win—and a huge blow to Houston Methodist who instigated COVID shot mandates—it still leaves our students vulnerable. Two years later, I am still writing exemptions for nursing students and hospital volunteers who are told they must take the COVID shots to participate in hospitals.

In a weak attempt to counter state lawmakers, Houston's mayor declared October 25—the day the Texas COVID-19 Vaccine Freedom Act passed—"Dr. Peter J. Hotez Day." I hope history remembers it instead as "COVID Vaccine Freedom Day," when David struck Goliath in Texas. The Texas medical establishment is probably bigger than Goliath but clearly not invincible.

Houston, a hub for COVID shot mandates, has also been at the center of transgender health controversies. General Surgeon Dr. Eithan Haim, a recent Baylor College of Medicine graduate, was indicted after exposing Texas Children's Hospital for continuing gender reassignment procedures on minors, despite assurances to Attorney General Ken Paxton and the public that it had ceased. Days later, nurse Vanessa Sivadge, another whistleblower, revealed the hospital's transgender clinic was fraudulently billing Medicaid, alleging providers used falsified diagnostic codes to get the government to pay for the services. Known as "miscoding" or "upcoding," providers have used incorrect billing codes to secure insurance coverage for services that would otherwise be denied. As the services they were providing violated SB 14, a Texas law prohibiting gender-affirming care for minors, diagnoses like "endocrine disorder," "testosterone deficiency," and "precocious puberty" were used instead.[1]

The outcry from state politicians was immediate and caught the attention of Attorney General Paxton, who swiftly stepped in, declaring he was launching an investigation into Texas Children's Hospital. The hospital retreated, taking down its press contact page, calling the cops on a reporter, and scrubbing their website's information of the two doctors implicated in the scandal, Drs. Richard Ogden Roberts and David Paul, as well as their entire board of directors.

The response from our elected officials was appropriate and expedient, but at the same time frustrating. The COVID response from our leaders has been far more tentative. Five years later, we are still trying to right the ship. No one has been held accountable, very few politicians will acknowledge the COVID shots are dangerous and should be pulled off the market, and the first hospital in the country to mandate the shots has yet to lose a lawsuit. Like a smoldering burn that will not extinguish, I continue to fight the Texas Medical Board to clear my name. I did not secretly insert hormone pellets into twelve-year-old girls and bill the taxpayers. Instead, I stepped on the toes of two multibillion dollar "nonprofit" hospitals by speaking up against mandates and fighting to protect—through the court system—the medical wishes of a dying man whose inpatient medical team refused to respect his rights.

COVID opened my eyes to a very dark side of healthcare, a side I had seen hints of throughout my career but had managed to avoid. When I moved from California to Texas, I assumed I was moving toward more freedom, but the blowback I and other physicians in Texas have received during the pandemic has challenged that assumption.

Thankfully, the DOJ dropped its case against Dr. Haim once Trump took office. Texas Children's Hospital's retaliation against Dr. Eithan Haim was harsher than my own experience, as I never faced potential prison time—likely a reflection of the intense ideological fervor he challenged. Both of us were thrust into the public eye and punished by authorities for upholding the Hippocratic Oath against extreme healthcare policies. Many wonder how such persecution could occur in seemingly conservative Texas, but I believe these attacks are orchestrated as part of a broader agenda. Healthcare is being used as a Trojan horse to advance far left ideologies and reshape Texas's political landscape. Vaccine mandates were just the start. Extremists knew that if they could enforce them in Texas, they could do so anywhere. As Texas goes, so goes the nation.

I live in Harris County, the most populous county in Texas, the third most populous county in the nation, and home to the largest medical complex in the world—the Texas Medical Center (TMC). The TMC hosts over sixty medical institutions, including the world's largest children's hospital (Texas Children's Hospital) and the world's largest cancer hospital (MD Anderson Cancer Center). I've wondered what sort of impact this gigantic system has on Texas state politics and decided to dig into the numbers.

Over the last ten years, Texas's population has surged. Austin's population has grown 33 percent, while Dallas and Houston have each grown 20 percent.[2] Recent figures show that, from 2021 to

2022, hundreds of thousands of people fled the blue cities of New York, Los Angeles, and Chicago to settle in Houston and Dallas.[3]

At the current rate, Texas expects to grow to approximately 2.3 million jobs by 2030, an 18.3 percent growth rate from 2020.[4] And where are these people working? In 2025, the top employment sector in Texas is healthcare.[5] Presently, the top position advertised online in Texas is for registered nurses.

Houston's Texas Medical Center (TMC) is the world's largest medical complex by several measures—number of hospitals, number of physicians, square footage, and patient volume. The TMC employs over 120,000 people, hosts ten million patient encounters annually, and has a gross domestic product of $25 billion.[6] Overall, the healthcare industry contributed over $161 billion to Texas's GDP in the last quarter of 2024.[7]

Over the past ten years, Texas grew its physician workforce at a faster rate than the state's population; the total number of physicians grew at 2.5 times the population rate.[8] Every year, nearly 2500 first year residents enter Texas to work in teaching hospitals, and this number is growing.[9] From 2021 to 2022, the number of newly licensed physicians increased by 1,300 (24 percent), from 5,300 newly licensed in 2021 to 6,600 newly licensed in 2022. This is the second highest year-over-year numerical increase for newly licensed physicians in Texas in forty years.[10]

The politics of the healthcare industry is moving left. In the last eight years, political action committee (PAC) contributions from health professionals to candidates have shifted allegiances. In 2014, the majority of contributions went to Republican candidates, but over the ensuing ten years, healthcare PACs have moved their money more to the Democrats.[11]

The Texas Medical Association (TMA) is the nation's largest medical society and claims to be the strongest voice for physicians in Texas. With over fifty-nine thousand members, approximately

80 percent of Texas physicians belong to the TMA. In 2022, they collected over $16 million in membership dues. Historically, TMA has been pro-physician and pro-patient, a group designed to help individual and small groups of doctors and their patients stand up against large hospitals and insurance companies. Lately, however, their public health policies, legislative priorities, candidate endorsements, and donor lists suggest otherwise.

Since 2010, the majority of funds raised by the TMA have supported Republicans, but in 2024, over 50 percent of donations went to Democrats, including vaccine crusaders and mandate enthusiasts Reps. Julie Johnson and Jasmine Crockett.[12] The two biggest line items on the TMA foundation's "Program Service Accomplishments" in 2022 were "Diversity and Medicine Scholarship" for $179,514 and "Vaccine Defend What Matters" for $106,021.[13]

Dr. Jimmy Widmer, head of TEXPAC, the political arm of the Texas Medical Association, testified against the Texas COVID-19 Vaccine Freedom Act and SB 177, a bill allowing individuals to reject the COVID-19 shots based on informed consent. Pediatrician and TMA activist Dr. Valerie Smith wrote opposing testimony to Texas Senate Bill 29, prohibiting government vaccine mandates, mask requirements, or private business or school closures to prevent the spread of COVID-19. In a TV interview, Dr. Smith recommended universal masking in schools.

TMA has written policies supporting universal flu vaccines[14] and removing parents' right to refuse vaccinations for their children.[15]

35.013 Universal Influenza Vaccination
'he Texas Medical Association supports the concept and goal of influenza vaccination for all individual
ix months and older except those with known contraindications (CPH Rep. 1-1-05; amended CSPH Rep
-A-15).

35.029 Restricting School Immunization Exemptions to Exemptions for Medical Reasons
'he Texas Medical Association advocates for the removal through legislation of nonmedical exemption
rom vaccinations approved and recommended by the Advisory Committee on Immunization Practices
ACIP) (Res. 350 2021).

At their annual meeting on May 5, 2024, Dr. Ori Hampel, a urologist in Houston, proposed a policy opposing mandates for any and all medical interventions. The overwhelming majority of the five hundred TMA delegates voted this measure down. The significance is profound. The largest medical association in the country believes the Texas government should retain the right to force its citizens to undergo a medical intervention.

SB 14, prohibiting gender transitioning procedures and treatments for minors, passed and was signed into law in 2023—but was opposed by TMA. Claiming to represent all fifty-five thousand physicians in Texas, Dr. Linda Villarreal, president of the Texas Medical Association, and Dr. Charleta Guillory, president of Texas Pediatric Society, sent a letter to Attorney General Paxton opposing "the criminalization of evidence-based, gender-affirming care for transgender youth and adolescents."[16]

TMA's policy outlining gender-affirming care for minors was crafted in 2021 by a small coalition of LGBQT activists—Drs. Brett Cooper, Shanna Combs, Emily Briggs, and Maria Monge. The language of their gender-affirming care policy is purposely confusing but amounts to supporting gender transitioning through medical interventions in minors and opposing therapy that might change their mind, known as "conversion therapy."

One of TMA's strongest proponents of transitioning minors is Dr. Maria Monge. Until recently, she was the director of adolescent medicine at Dell Children's Medical Center in Austin, Texas, but departed after Attorney General Paxton announced an investigation into the hospital for illegal performance of gender transitioning procedures on minors. Of note, every doctor in the adolescent medicine department at Dell Children's Medical Center left the hospital following Paxton's announcement.

Dr. Monge honed her strong views on gender-affirming care during her training at Boston Children's adolescent care program.

She now operates an independent practice in Austin. A source close to her shared that she is deeply committed to providing gender-affirming care.

In 2021, the Texas Medical Association passed a resolution opposing the criminalization of gender-affirming treatments for minors. A former TMA leader revealed that medical students were used as a Trojan horse to advance this policy. Despite representing only twelve of the five hundred delegates, the medical student section submitted forty resolutions last session. Audio obtained from a former TMA board member during a January 28, 2022, LGBTQ section meeting attended by Drs. Brett Cooper, Sealy Massingill, Shanna Combs, Emily Briggs, and John Carlo revealed how a small group of activists strategically pushed controversial policies. Dr. Massingill, chief medical officer (CMO) of Planned Parenthood, stated, "We need the right Trojan horse to bring that in... Shanna [Combs], just putting the text isn't the worst idea, but finding the right Trojan horse would be easier and less problematic." The group deliberately had medical students introduce the policy to avoid pushback that would have arisen if it came directly from the LGBTQ section.

Doe v. Abbott is a lawsuit brought by a family investigated by the Texas Department of Family and Protective Services (DFPS). Governor Greg Abbott issued a directive on February 22, 2022, ordering the Texas Department of Family and Protective Services (DFPS) to investigate parents providing gender-affirming care to their transgender children as potential child abuse. In response, Texas Children's Hospital, once touting itself as the "preeminent, top-tier transgender medical program in the US,"[17] paused their program, and the parents of a transitioning child who were investigated sued. Texas Medical Association filed a friend-of-the-court brief in support of the plaintiffs (March 10, 2022): "TMA supports physician efforts to provide medically appropriate therapies relating to gender identity and opposes the criminalization of these practices."[18] The lawsuit is pending appeal before the Third Court of Appeals.

Doe v. Abbott is backed by Lambda Legal, the ACLU, and the law firm of Baker Botts. Lambda Legal was started in 1971 to advocate for gay rights. The firm has grown to thirty attorneys, and due to his known ties to the ACLU, some suspect George Soros is a key financial supporter. With assets estimated over $54 million,[19] Lambda Legal has expanded to become active in transgender cases, notably ones involving minors. Another minor gender modification case they were involved in, *Loe v. Texas*,[20] challenging SB 14, was shut down by the Supreme Court of Texas on June 28, 2024.

During the TMA annual meeting in 2024, Dr. D. Michael Ready, a family practitioner in Temple, Texas, submitted a proposal to change the language of TMA's guidelines from "gender-affirming care" to "evidenced-based care." Of all the resolutions proposed, this one stimulated the most pushback, inciting a storm of LGBTQ TMA activists to submit written testimony in opposition. His efforts really didn't stand a chance—nearly 80 percent of the five hundred delegates voted against this resolution, and it was swiftly struck down.

Dr. M. Brett Cooper, Assistant Professor in the Department of Pediatrics at UT Southwestern Medical Center, is a specialist in adolescent medicine, including puberty consultations and LGBTQ health, and has served as an expert witness for the Texas Medical Board as well as testified to lawmakers on behalf of the TMA. In November 2024, Texas Attorney General Paxton filed a lawsuit against Dr. Cooper for allegedly violating the Texas law banning gender-affirming care for minors. The lawsuit, filed in Collin County District Court, accuses Cooper of prescribing testosterone to fifteen biologically female minors, aged fourteen to seventeen, for gender transition purposes after the ban took effect on September

1, 2023. Paxton's office claims Cooper falsified medical records, using diagnoses like "precocious puberty" or "endocrine disorder" to conceal gender dysphoria treatments, and seeks $10,000 in civil penalties per violation, a temporary injunction, and revocation of Cooper's medical license. Paxton filed similar lawsuits against Cooper's colleague at UT Southwestern, Dr. May Lau, and another physician in El Paso, Dr. Hector Granados. All three have been barred from practicing medicine while their lawsuits proceed. On February 28, 2025, Judge Christine Nowak of the 493rd District Court denied Cooper's and Lau's motions to dismiss, allowing the cases to proceed.

Attorney General Ken Paxton is the first in the country to prosecute physicians for violating laws against gender transition of minors, but Texas is not the only state with these laws—and it wasn't the first. Arkansas paved the way, enacting the first ban on all gender transitioning of minors in 2021, with the legislature overriding a veto from Governor Asa Hutchinson.[21] Twenty-seven states have enacted similar laws, but over half of these bans face legal challenges, with Arkansas's ban permanently blocked and Montana's temporarily blocked. SCOTUS recently upheld Tennessee's ban on gender transitioning of minors and will likely set a precedent for other states. On the flip side, sixteen states have implemented "shield laws" to protect physicians providing hormones and surgery to minors wishing to change their sex.

Despite the Texas law, TMA offered a CME course on transgender practices at their annual meeting on May 5th, 2024. Activists Brett Cooper, Emily Briggs, and Sealy Massingill were part of the team that presented this talk. The talk included material on adolescents and children, including the "Genderbread Person" and the "Gender Unicorn."

In addition to supporting medical mandates and transitioning minors, the TMA opposes physician free speech. In 2023, the

TMA Board of Trustees created a "medical disinformation" policy. Witnesses claim my name was brought up multiple times during the meeting drafting this policy. The ringleaders for this resolution were pediatricians Dr. Jason Terk and Dr. Valerie Smith—both members of TMA's COVID-19 Task Force. Dr. Terk, a member of TMA's Committee for Science and Public Health for the past two years, reportedly targeted me and other physicians who publicly opposed mandates.

As a member of the censorship group "Shots Heard Round the World," TMA was part of an online effort encouraging the public to report me and other physicians to the medical boards. TMA member and Houston pediatrician Dr. Christina Propst spurred other members to make fake claims against me to the Texas Medical Board, posting to the group: "Short on time so sharing some screenshots about a Houston medspa/cosmetic ENT and her egregious cash-only COVID profiteering and COVID misinformation spreading bullshittery that has persisted throughout the pandemic. She's a local cash-only sketchy COVID test and Ivermectin queen."

After including the link to report me to the Texas Medical Board, she added instructions on what to accuse me of. "Entering the demographic info for her practice is [sic] literally takes a minute so I included it in a screenshot below. The rest is easy peasy. Reason: 1- Unprofessional Conduct (aka spreading COVID Misinformation), 2- Quality of Care/Prescribing. Put yourself as the "Person/Patient Harmed."

I reported this action of Dr. Propst to the medical board, but the Board declined to investigate, admitting they don't regulate speech. Their decision letter is on the following page.

When I posted evidence of TMA's membership in "Shots Heard Round the World" on X, TMA responded by blocking me. I've sent them numerous emails asking for an explanation. All have

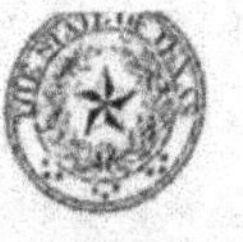

Texas Medical Board

September 29, 2023

MARY BOWDEN

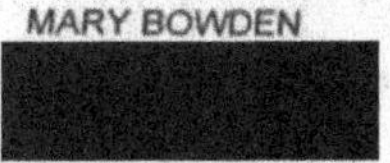

Re: File #24-0324 PROPST

Dear MS BOWDEN

Your complaint has been reviewed to determine if a licensee of this agency is involved and whether a state law or board rule has been violated. As you know, the Texas Medical Board enforces those requirements governing the practice of medicine as set forth in the Texas Occupations Code and board rules.

The Texas Medical Board does not regulate speech, as such based on the information available to the Board. there is no violation of the Medical Practice Act or Board Rules, and no further action will be taken.

Sincerely,

The Texas Medical Board

remained unanswered. I still continue to pay them $810 in annual dues to preserve my TMLT malpractice insurance.

TMA and TMLT share a close relationship, with TMLT holding a near-monopoly on medical malpractice insurance in Texas, facilitated by TMA. A former Board member of TMA told me TMA blocks TMLT competitors from exhibiting at its annual meeting, allegedly denying MedPro a booth—despite MedPro offering TMA $1 million to advertise at the meeting—and similarly excluding other insurers. Additionally, TMLT requires TMA membership as a condition of coverage. Dr. Joseph Valenti, chair of TMA's Board of Trustees, was overheard celebrating this mandate, describing it as "golden handcuffs" for Texas physicians.

Dr. Valenti serves on the board of both TMLT and TMA. Practicing as a gynecologist, Valenti is a regular donor to Democrats and is particularly fond of Rep. Julie Johnson, a very vocal abortion activist in Texas.

As Texas does not have a state surgeon general, Governor Abbott relied on Texas Department of State Health Services (DSHS) Commissioner Dr. John Hellerstedt during the pandemic, who spoke of his close relationship with TMA. "We had daily discussions with TMA," in coordination with the association's COVID-19 Task Force, he reflected. "They were a great resource for getting out information to other physicians. It was extremely helpful to have that [coordination] and be able to have regular in-depth conversations with medical professionals."[22] Prior to his DSHS term, Dr. Hellerstedt served as a consultant to TMA's Council on Public Health.

Dr. Hellerstedt was eventually awarded with the Texas Hospital Association's THA Trustee Award—the highest honor given to someone not directly involved in hospital management. The THA commended him for "wearing a mask and becoming one of the first Texans to become vaccinated against COVID-19.... During industry-wide calls to address the pandemic, Dr. Hellerstedt made sure the needs of hospitals were amplified as the state public health team worked to respond."[23] Dr. Marc Boom, CEO of Houston Methodist Hospital, helped present his award.

Current Texas DSHS Commissioner, Dr. Jennifer Shuford, who was front and center during TMA's COVID Task Force meetings, spoke of the chemistry between TMA and the public health agency: "TMA has been an extraordinary partner during my time as commissioner."[24] Shuford served as consultant to TMA's Council of

Science and Public Health and Committee on Infectious Diseases and recently attended TMA's leadership conference in January to address the state's syphilis epidemic.

"The benefit is mutual, and I can say that having been a member of TMA before [becoming commissioner]. Seeing everything that they can do to improve the lives of patients through public health is great ... I had no idea they [TMA] were such an advocate for public health until I was in this role." [25]

Texas has become a testing ground for far-left public health policies, with healthcare dominated by a professional organization that supports vaccine mandates, gender transitioning of minors, and physician censorship. I believe Houston Methodist was deliberately chosen—five months before Biden's federal mandate—as the first US hospital to mandate COVID vaccines. By implementing mandates in the largest Republican, freedom-loving state, Houston Methodist demonstrated mandates could succeed anywhere. Targeting me, a solo physician insignificant to their revenue, sent a clear warning to other doctors who might consider speaking out. TMA played a key role in this effort. TMA should be dismantled, and its close ties to the state's largest malpractice insurance carrier warrant an antitrust investigation.

CHAPTER 17

Hospital Murders

During the pandemic, my primary focus was managing outpatients, but I had several hospitalized patients, like Jason Jones, reach out for help, and reviewed numerous charts for families seeking answers after losing loved ones. I've heard countless stories from patients, colleagues, and nurses about their hospital experiences across different facilities. Despite the varied settings, these accounts share striking similarities.

Upon entering the hospital, COVID patients faced immediate physical isolation. They rarely saw or were examined by physicians, raising concerns about informed consent. Nurses provided most of the care, often serving as the patients' sole human contact. This hospital-enforced solitary confinement harmed patients' physical recovery, mental health, and social well-being, with lasting effects persisting beyond their hospital stays.

A 2020 *Critical Care* journal analysis found that isolated ICU patients had higher rates of ventilator-associated pneumonia due to reduced staff oversight.[1] Isolation often disrupted meal assistance, leading to inadequate caloric intake, particularly in elderly patients. A 2022 *Journal of Clinical Nursing* study reported that isolated patients consumed about 15 percent less food on average, contributing to weight loss and slower recovery.[2] A 2020 *Psychiatry Research* study found that 53 percent of isolated COVID patients showed moderate-to-severe anxiety, compared to 30 percent in non-isolated patients.[3] Lack of family visits and restricted staff interaction worsened feelings of loneliness. Particularly in ICUs, sensory deprivation from familiar faces and routines increased delirium risk. A 2020 *JAMA Neurology* report noted a 65 percent higher delirium incidence in isolated elderly patients versus non-isolated peers, linked to cognitive decline post-discharge.[4] Prolonged isolation correlated with PTSD symptoms. A 2022 *Lancet* study estimated that about 20 percent of isolated COVID survivors showed PTSD symptoms six months post-discharge, tied to feelings of helplessness and lack of control.[5]

The impact on family members when loved ones died alone in hospitals during COVID, due to isolation protocols, was profound. Family members often experienced overwhelming guilt for not being present at the time of death. A 2021 *Journal of Pain and Symptom Management* study found that 63 percent of bereaved relatives whose loved ones died alone in hospitals reported "complicated grief," characterized by persistent yearning and inability to accept the loss, compared to 40 percent for non-isolated deaths.[6] Witnessing a loved one's decline remotely (via video, for example) or receiving abrupt death notifications without closure increased trauma. A 2022 *Frontiers in Psychiatry* study estimated that 25 percent of these family members showed PTSD symptoms, linked to the abruptness and isolation of the death.[7] Prolonged grief disorder was more common, with a 2022 *The Lancet Psychiatry* study estimating that 15 percent of these families met diagnostic criteria a year later, compared to 8 percent for non-COVID bereavements.[8]

Many developed skepticism toward medical institutions. A 2021 *Social Science & Medicine* survey found that 40 percent of affected families reported reduced trust in hospitals.[9]

Patients and families had limited say in their treatments, and most doctors relied on government-dictated protocols with poor outcomes. Monoclonal antibodies were incredibly effective and very safe, but since the FDA restricted EUA of monoclonal antibodies for outpatients, the moment a patient crossed the threshold of the hospital, their opportunity to receive monoclonal antibodies was over. Even as an outpatient, they were difficult to obtain, as many physicians rationed their use to people considered high risk. New York, Utah, and Minnesota implemented guidelines that considered race and ethnicity as factors in prioritizing who was eligible to receive monoclonal antibody treatments.

The drug of choice for COVID patients in the ICU, Remdesivir, was fraught with problems. A 2020 study reported 23 percent of patients on Remdesivir experienced increased hepatic enzymes,[10] and acute kidney injury occurred in 10 to 25 percent of patients with at least one comorbidity. Some studies have shown it shortens recovery time in hospitalized patients,[11] but multiple studies have failed to find any mortality benefit.[12,13]

Though not clinically effective, Remdesivir was financially lucrative for hospitals. From November 2, 2020, to September 30, 2023, the Centers for Medicare & Medicaid Services (CMS) provided an additional payment of up to 65 percent of the drug's cost (approximately $2,028 for a $3,120 course) for Medicare patients, on top of the standard DRG payment. For inpatient stays with a primary or secondary diagnosis of COVID-19, Medicare increased the DRG payment by 20 percent over the standard amount (DRG, "diagnosis-related group" is a Medicare payment system that categorizes inpatient hospital stays based on diagnoses, procedures, and patient characteristics to determine standardized reimbursement amounts for hospitals).

I reviewed hospital charts for many families whose loved ones died from COVID. Commonly, patients received inadequate doses of inappropriate steroids, were denied breathing treatments due to concerns about viral spread, and were given potent diuretics to reduce lung fluid. Concurrently, hospitals restricted fluids and nutrition, often causing severe dehydration and malnutrition. The combination of diuretics, fluid restriction, and the nephrotoxic drug Remdesivir placed significant strain on the kidneys, potentially leading to kidney failure, even in patients without preexisting renal conditions.

A tragic case I reviewed for a family still haunts me. John Nelson Russell, an eighteen-year-old healthy boy from Houston, went to the Memorial Hermann Hospital ER with COVID and an oxygen saturation of 84 percent. His lab results showed he was dehydrated with severely elevated muscle enzymes, indicative of rhabdomyolysis, a condition that requires vigorous hydration. Instead, the doctor ordered "cautious IV hydration with normal saline at 50cc/hr." He asked for a Gatorade, and the nurse told him no. He received Remdesivir, went into kidney failure, and died.

Morphine is often administered to terminally ill patients nearing death to alleviate pain and dyspnea, a practice known as "comfort care." This is permissible, provided the intent is to relieve suffering, not to hasten death. Euthanasia, by contrast, involves administering medication to intentionally end life. While the distinction can be nuanced, providers treating terminally ill patients who decline further intervention are generally afforded discretion, assuming their actions prioritize patient comfort.

Morphine, primarily used for pain relief, is frequently administered in the ICU to alleviate shortness of breath, but it requires careful titration due to the risk of respiratory depression, as morphine suppresses the brain's respiratory drive. In COVID patients with acute respiratory distress, reduced lung compliance heightens the danger of morphine's respiratory effects. A 2020 study in the *American Journal of Respiratory and Critical Care Medicine* found that morphine increased mortality risk in patients with respiratory distress when not carefully titrated.[14]

Morphine is commonly used in ICUs to alleviate suffering, and providers rarely face judgment when critically ill patients die, provided their intent is palliative. Dr. Anna Pou, one of my attending physicians during residency, was investigated by Louisiana Attorney General Charles Foti for administering lethal morphine doses to ICU patients at Memorial Medical Center after Hurricane Katrina caused prolonged power outages. Autopsies confirmed morphine contributed to the deaths of nine ICU patients, with four deaths showing signs of human intervention, implicating Dr. Pou. In 2007, charges were dropped, and Dr. Pou was exonerated, as investigators determined she acted in good faith to provide comfort under extreme circumstances.[15]

Physicians exercise great caution when administering morphine to critically ill patients in respiratory distress, especially those without a Do Not Resuscitate (DNR) order, a directive prohibiting cardiopulmonary resuscitation (CPR) or other lifesaving measures during cardiac or respiratory arrest. Based on my review of numerous hospital charts from the pandemic, I suspect some providers may have blurred the line between comfort care and euthanasia in their use of morphine, potentially hiding inappropriate intent.

A patient of mine asked me to review her brother's chart following his unexpected death at a hospital in McAllen, Texas. He was fifty years old and otherwise healthy. When he fell ill with COVID, he developed shortness of breath and went to the hospital. His hospital course was typical of many others. He was isolated, fluid-restricted, minimally nourished, and subjected to a protocol-driven treatment plan that ended in his death.

His chart was over two thousand pages long, but careful scrutiny of the minutes surrounding his death revealed shocking information. Despite a pain score of "0," a respiratory rate of three breaths/minute and a blood glucose of 127 mg/dL, his physician ordered morphine and insulin; the patient died four minutes later. He was a full code, no DNR, and was not diabetic.

The administration of morphine to a patient with a respiratory rate of three, barely sustaining life, suggests the physician and nurse intended to hasten death, as morphine's respiratory depression would likely accelerate the inevitable outcome. Similarly, the insulin administration appeared nontherapeutic. Critically ill ICU patients often develop hyperglycemia, managed with insulin via a sliding scale protocol, where doses are adjusted based on blood glucose levels, typically starting at 150 mg/dL. Administering insulin to a near-death patient with a near-normal glucose level deviates significantly from standard practice.

I reported the doctor to the Texas Medical Board and reported the incident to the McAllen police department. The Medical Board sent me a letter stating that, after their own preliminary investigation, they were not going to take the investigation any further. I never heard back from the McAllen police department.

At the time this patient was fighting for his life in McAllen, Texas, a young woman in Wisconsin was engaged in a similar battle. Like many hospitalized patients during the pandemic, half of her struggles entailed fighting the system charged with saving her.

In October 2021, Grace Schara, a nineteen-year-old with Down syndrome, died at St. Elizabeth Hospital in Wisconsin under tragic circumstances. Her death highlights a disturbing convergence of hospital protocols, medical negligence, and systemic failures during the pandemic. Allegations of intentional misconduct led to a groundbreaking lawsuit, the first of its kind to reach a jury trial.

Grace, described by her father, Scott, as a "gift from God," contracted COVID in September 2021. Initially, the Schara family followed the Front Line COVID-19 Critical Care Alliance (FLCCC) protocol, using ivermectin and vitamins. However, a critical decision to purchase a pulse oximeter, driven by pandemic propaganda, proved fatal. When Grace's oxygen saturation dropped to 88 percent, the family, adhering to protocol recommendations, admitted her to the hospital on October 6, 2021. Scott later reflected that this reliance on a number, without a baseline or understanding of oxygen saturation, was a grave mistake. Grace might still be alive had they not sought hospital care.

Once admitted, Grace's condition stabilized on simple oxygen. Despite this, hospital staff quickly escalated her treatment to high-flow oxygen devices and BiPAP (bilevel positive airway pressure), often without clear communication to Scott, who was present as her advocate. On October 10, Scott was forcibly removed from the hospital by an armed guard, accused of having COVID symptoms and interfering with care. During the forty-seven hours Grace was without an advocate, the staff administered Precedex, a potent IV sedative drip, increasing its dosage six times until reaching the maximum amount permitted. On October 13, while Grace's sister Jessica was briefly absent, the hospital restrained Grace, leading to her defecating in bed. That same day, Dr. Gavin Shokar placed an unauthorized Do Not Resuscitate (DNR) order on her chart. The family did not preapprove authorization for intubation, but they never authorized or signed a Do Not Intubate or Do Not Resuscitate order. As a family member was with her, they wanted to decide as the situation arose.

The sequence of events on Grace's final day is chilling. Between 10:48 a.m. and 6:15 p.m., staff administered a maximum dose of

Precedex, three doses of lorazepam, and morphine—medications with compounded sedative side effects and akin to hospice euthanasia protocols. Despite Scott questioning the morphine, the doctor claimed it was to "slow her breathing." By 7:18 p.m., Grace's vitals plummeted while her sister Jessica, on a FaceTime call with her parents, pleaded for help. For ten minutes, Jessica insisted there was no DNR, but the nurses refused to intervene. Grace died at 7:27 p.m. as her family watched helplessly.

The Schara family's lawsuit, filed in April 2023, named Dr. Shokar and nurses Alison Barkholtz and Hollee McInnis, alleging medical malpractice and battery due to the unauthorized DNR and intentional administration of lethal medications. Attorney Warner Mendenhall emphasized the battery claim, which holds individuals personally liable, bypassing protections like the PREP (Public Readiness and Emergency Preparedness) Act. The case, one of the first COVID-related lawsuits to reach a jury trial, faced challenges, including Wisconsin's $750,000 medical malpractice cap, which deters attorneys from taking such cases. Yet, the Scharas did not seek financial gain; awards were intended to support Grace's nonprofit to raise awareness.

Discovery revealed systemic issues—doctors adhering to rigid protocols, ignoring patient needs, and a lack of accountability. Notably, Grace's medical records labeled her a "non-VIP patient," suggesting differential treatment, possibly exacerbated by her unvaccinated status and Down Syndrome. The case highlights broader discrimination against vulnerable populations, including the elderly and disabled, during the pandemic.

The trial recently ended with the jury ruling in favor of the hospital eleven to one. As deliberations lasted less than an hour, the jury likely had their minds made up and didn't review the evidence. A DNR requires a signature and a witness and can be verbally reversed at any time, but the jury absolved the doctor and nurses of all wrongdoing. The loss sets an alarming precedent, essentially authorizing hospitals to make patients' DNR orders without consent and condoning euthanasia. To learn more about Grace, please visit the website in her honor, www.ourAmazingGrace.net. To donate to the foundation set up in her name, please visit www.givesendgo.com/theskysthelimit.

In the press conference following the verdict, attorney Mendenhall stated, "When you go into a hospital, you sign your rights away."[16] The frightening reality of this case is that Grace had a very supportive family advocating for her, yet she still fell victim to hospital abuse. Everyone should be prepared before going to the hospital—understand your rights and designate in writing what you do and do not consent to. In response to almost succumbing to hospital protocols, my friend Greta Crawford started a website called "Protocol Kills" that educates the public about their hospital rights. She and Laura Bartlett created a template patients can fill out in advance, designating COVID-specific treatments. Visit www.protocolkills.com for more information.

Author's note on sources for this chapter:

I wrote this chapter June 2025 and submitted it to Post Hill Press on June 24, 2025. When I received comments from the editor on August 19, 2025, I was alarmed to find five of the sources I cited in this chapter have been entirely removed from the internet (see endnotes throughout this chapter). Even after checking Wayback Machine, Grok, and Retraction Watch, I have been unable to find these articles. All five of these articles concern harmful hospital practices during the pandemic.

CHAPTER 18

Federation of State Medical Boards

The suppression of dissent in favor of orthodoxy, a practice rooted in ancient times, persists today, as physicians who challenged prevailing narratives during the pandemic faced significant professional repercussions. Just as Galileo faced the Inquisition for his astronomical assertions, pandemic physicians and scientists like myself encountered massive institutional pushback when our views diverged from government doctrines.

Many of us across the country have had to defend ourselves against medical boards after voicing concerns about vaccines, fighting mask mandates, and prescribing ivermectin. During the Texas mask mandate instituted by Governor Greg Abbott, the Texas Medical Board temporarily suspended the license of fellow ENT Dr. Eric Hensen after a patient turned him in for not wearing a mask in his office. Elsewhere in Texas, Drs. Richard Urso, Joe Varon, and Stella Immanuel have had to defend themselves against prescribing hydroxychloroquine and ivermectin for COVID patients. All of us who have come under attack from the Texas Medical Board during the pandemic are still licensed, but the stress and expense of defending ourselves has been enormous.

The entity behind these accusations, the Federation of State Medical Boards (FSMB), directed state medical boards to enforce policies promoting COVID vaccination and mask mandates. Though a private institution, FSMB is somehow able to exercise coercive control over government-run medical boards through threats of disciplinary measures. Pursuant to the FSMB's bylaws, "[t]he Board of Directors, on behalf of the House of Delegates, may enforce disciplinary measures, including expulsion, suspension, censure and reprimand" against a member Medical Board.[1]

Over the past decades, FSMB has taken over many of the traditional examination, database, credentialing, and regulatory functions of state medical boards. FSMB maintains an extensive "Public Policy Compendium," with various resolutions, reports, position statements, model regulations, and other quasi-legislative material containing various degrees of binding language addressed toward state medical boards and physicians, including terms like "required to," "encouraged to," "have a responsibility to," "recommended to," "urged to," "should," and "must."

Together with the National Board of Medical Examiners, FSMB operates the United States Medical Licensing Examination (USMLE), which replaced traditional state board examinations and is mandatory for all US medical school graduates seeking licensure. The USMLE generates significant revenue for FSMB, which reported $70,524,058 in tax-exempt income in 2024, with the largest share from the USMLE ($35,810,735.)[2]

This financial and regulatory clout underpins the FSMB's ability to enforce medical orthodoxy, as seen during the pandemic. On July 15, 2021, Surgeon General Vivek Murthy declared medical misinformation a public health emergency, issuing a call to arms to social media companies to censor its users. Two weeks later, on

July 29, 2021, the FSMB issued a press release warning doctors that spreading pandemic-related misinformation could lead to disciplinary action, including license revocation. That same day, Biden announced federal employees must disclose their vaccination status, with the unvaccinated subject to special restrictions.

The FSMB's warning against medical misinformation, issued alongside federal mandates, set the stage for a broader campaign to enforce compliance among physicians. On September 9, 2021, the American Board of Internal Medicine (ABIM), American Board of Family Medicine (ABFM), and American Board of Pediatrics (ABP) emailed physicians nationwide, endorsing the FSMB's stance that spreading misinformation could lead to loss of medical license or board certification. This email coincided with President Biden's announcement that employers with one hundred or more employees must mandate COVID-19 vaccinations.

This coordinated institutional pressure swiftly impacted my case. On December 13, 2021, the FDA sent a letter to the FSMB warning about physicians prescribing ivermectin. The next day, Houston Methodist Hospital reported me to the National Practitioner Data Bank (NPDB), and on December 22, 2021, I received notice of their complaint to the Texas Medical Board, which centered on my use of ivermectin.

The institutional campaign to enforce medical compliance, which fueled complaints against me over ivermectin, intensified with formal policy changes. In April 2022, the FSMB adopted a policy titled, "Professional Expectations Regarding Medical Misinformation and Disinformation," prohibiting licensed physicians from publishing or speaking about scientific evidence that contradicted consensus-driven dogma. This policy redefined "scientific evidence" as limited to peer-reviewed journals, methodologically sound clinical trials, nationally or internationally recognized clinical practice guidelines, or broadly accepted consensus-based documents, shifting the term from empirical data to textual authority.

This FSMB censorship policy forbids all licensed physicians in America from publicly expressing any medical opinions not based on the FSMB's definition of a consensus-based document. "When medical information is conveyed, whether in a clinical setting or in public through electronic means or otherwise, it must be based upon the best available scientific evidence.... If justification based on scientific evidence is not present, disciplinary action by a state medical board may be warranted."[3]

Misinformation is defined as medical or otherwise "[h]ealth-related information or claims that are false, inaccurate or misleading, according to the best available scientific evidence at the time." Disinformation is a sub-category of misinformation "that is spread intentionally to serve a malicious purpose, such as financial gain or political advantage."[4]

The FSMB Censorship Policy requires Member Medical Boards to adopt "a specific policy on misinformation ... in light of the increased prevalence of, and harm caused by, physician-disseminated misinformation in this ongoing pandemic.... When adjudicating cases regarding misinformation and disinformation, state medical boards are encouraged to consider the full array of authorized grounds for disciplinary action in their Medical Practice Acts.... State medical boards should not be dissuaded from carrying out their duty to protect the public by concerns about potential challenges to disciplinary decisions when these decisions are based on sound regulatory considerations for public protection."[5]

FSMB's House of Delegates approved the censorship policy after listening to a speech by the US Public Health Service Commissioned Corps's Admiral Rachel Levine on April 30, 2022, about "health misinformation." Admiral Levine complained to the FSMB delegates that health misinformation "has divided our nation," has "undermined vaccination efforts to defeat COVID-19," and undermined the belief that "the positive value of gender-affirming care for youth and adults is not in scientific or medical dispute."[6]

The FSMB's then-Chair asked Admiral Levine: "Can you offer any advice or guidance to state medical boards as we continue to manage complaints against our licensed providers who post COVID misinformation?"

Admiral Levine replied, "I think that it is something that is under the purview of the medical boards and I think that this meeting that you're having is maybe the perfect forum to discuss that issue.... [I] refer you to the Surgeon General's work on this issue and if you're interested, please contact my office. I'll be pleased to contact you with the Surgeon General because this is a specific issue that he is working on."

Under the section, "Legislative Interference with Medical Regulatory Boards," the FSMB's 2022 House of Delegates Annual Meeting Guidebook, which was given out to delegates at the meeting, describes the FSMB's aggressive fight on the side of censorship against the actual lawful regulators of medicine in the United States:

> An issue related to the pandemic has been the effort by state legislatures across the United States to undercut the authority of state medical boards' regulatory and disciplinary efforts. At least 20 pieces of legislation have been proposed in multiple states, in addition to two pieces of legislation that became law in 2021.
>
> (North Dakota and Tennessee), that would curtail the ability of state medical boards to investigate or discipline physicians who dispense FDA-approved drugs for off-label use in treating COVID-19 or who publicly discuss the treatment methods they use for COVID-19, which are not scientifically supported. Our advocacy team has been working diligently in

response, including providing direct testimony to state legislators about the harm of these efforts to patient safety.[7]

The FSMB significantly influenced state medical boards during the pandemic by enforcing a censorship policy that redefined scientific evidence as consensus-based, punishing physicians for dissenting views on vaccines, masks, or off-label treatments like ivermectin. Echoing Galileo's 1633 trial for challenging orthodoxy, physicians across the country faced investigations for noncompliance, incurring substantial stress and costs. The FSMB's coercive control, backed by millions of dollars in revenue and disciplinary authority over seventy member boards, stifled debate and eroded public trust, as seen in its opposition to legislative protections for physician autonomy.

The FSMB's actions have significantly chilled medical discourse. To protect medical dissent, restore trust, and ensure evidence-based practice free from institutional dogma, I have joined three other physicians in a lawsuit against the FSMB, medical boards, and their members. We allege violations of our First Amendment rights to challenge the prevailing scientific consensus and assert that the FSMB and defendants engaged in a conspiracy to restrain trade. Should they claim immunity from restraint of trade liability as government entities, such immunity would subject them to First Amendment liability.

CHAPTER 19

The Flaming Sword of Justice

During the peak of the pandemic, I juggled caring for the sick, raising my four children, and defending myself against attacks from an army of individuals and their institutions. When the Texas Medical Board and Houston Methodist targeted me, my first and only instinct was to fight back; to that goal, I have dedicated much of my free time to giving interviews, speaking at conferences, and sharing my perspectives on social media.

As the pandemic waned, my medical practice has shifted from treating acutely ill COVID patients to helping those with injuries from the COVID shots. As an ENT surgeon, I'm accustomed to fixing issues quickly, as most ear, nose, and throat conditions respond well to interventions—a key reason I chose this specialty. However, patients with vaccine-related injuries are quite challenging and recover slowly. With limited research, treatments often involve trial and error approaches, many of which are not covered by insurance, and incremental progress takes months rather than days.

I was hopeful Robert F. Kennedy Jr.'s appointment as HHS Secretary would be the lifeboat my patients and I have been looking for, but his position of power has not led to the pandemic-related reforms we expected. Backed by the Make America Healthy Again (MAHA) movement, Kennedy has pivoted from criticizing mRNA shots to tackling chronic childhood diseases, advocating for phasing out synthetic food dyes like FD&C Red No. 40, removing fluoride from our water, and collaborating with the USDA to restrict SNAP benefits for purchasing soda, candy, and unhealthy foods.

This shift was cemented in the seventy-six page "MAHA Report," released May 16, 2025,[1] which omitted any mention of mRNA. In a subsequent report, issued on September 9, 2025, MAHA provided a long list of environmental threats to our health, again with zero mention of mRNA.[2] The leaders of MAHA might think the threat of mRNA is trivial, assuming few people continue to get COVID shots, but during the September 2025 ACIP meeting (CDC's Advisory Committee on Immunization Practices), the CDC admitted large numbers of children continue to receive them, reporting approximately 13 percent of children six months to seventeen years of age, or 9.5 million children in America, received a COVID shot in 2024.[3]

Further, the push for injecting our population with mRNA is only just beginning. With five hundred mRNA products in the pipeline, the FDA recently approved Moderna's mNexspike COVID shot for public use, bypassing consultation with the Vaccines and Related Biological Products Advisory Committee (VRBPAC), and granted fast-track status to Arcturus's self-amplifying mRNA shot for H5N1. Moderna's mRESVIA mRNA vaccine against RSV was approved for adults May 31, 2024.[4]

Additionally, the agency approved a new RSV monoclonal antibody for newborns, despite a nearly four-fold increase in risk of seizures following the injection.[5] While Kennedy's HHS leadership has sidestepped mRNA concerns in favor of food-focused initiatives, in March 2025, the CDC made a modest adjustment to its pediatric vaccine schedule by replacing its recommendation of three mRNA shots by nine months with a "shared clinical decision-making" approach for children.[6] At the September 2025 ACIP meeting, members went further, expanding the "shared clinical decision-making" label for the COVID shot to all ages, including adults.

Going forward, the CDC no longer recommends the COVID shots for anyone but leaves the decision between a physician and the patient.[7] While this is a step in the right direction, given the current reality of the disease along with the demonstrated risks of the shots, the COVID shots should not be available to anyone. COVID has evolved into a mild upper respiratory infection, and while I once worried about my COVID patients, I now rarely see them in my office and no longer fear hospitalizations. The CDC's "shared clinical decision-making" approach feels more like a political compromise than a science-based policy, raising concerns that individuals with minimal risk factors will face pressure to receive these shots.

As Secretary of Health and Human Services, Robert F. Kennedy Jr. can implement significant changes without Congressional approval. The swine flu vaccine was halted in nine states in 1976 after just three deaths, and the RotaShield vaccine was withdrawn in 1999 after ten to fifteen cases of bowel obstruction. In contrast, the FDA continues to promote COVID shots, despite 38,615 reported deaths in VAERS and multiple data sources showing risks outweigh benefits. With the CDC's vaccination policies out of step with COVID's current mild nature, and the executive branch slow to act, attention has turned to legislators for solutions. Last session, nine states introduced bills to ban mRNA vaccines, but none advanced past a hearing. In Texas, seven bills—four for humans (House Bills

3737 and 3465 by Rep. Joanne Shofner, HB 3176 by freshman Rep. Wesley Virdell, and HB 5022 by Rep. Helen Kerwin) and three for animals (Senate Bills 1887 by Sen. Kevin Sparks and SB 1983 and SB 119 by Sen. Bob Hall)—gained broad support, with twenty-four of the eighty-eight Republican House legislators (27 percent) co-sponsoring at least one. However, all but one bill stalled, as House Committee on Public Health Chair Rep. Gary VanDeaver ignored them, leaving the four House bills without even a committee hearing.

Despite the failure of legislators to advance mRNA bans, my organization, Americans for Health Freedom, is building a growing list of politicians willing to publicly demand the removal of COVID shots from the market. Though this list expands daily, it represents only a small fraction of elected officials. The widespread silence from those entrusted to protect us is profoundly disappointing. I am certain most officials have privately rejected CDC recommendations, refusing mRNA shots for themselves and their children, yet they stay quiet, allowing constituents to face risks they personally are unwilling to take.

The last recourse when our elected officials won't act is to turn to the legal system. Though costly and time-intensive, the courtroom is the only option for change when the executive and legislative branches fail to act. Before the pandemic, I had no experience in this realm, but I've since gained more insight than I care to know into the legalities of public health policy.

My crash immersion in law required confronting the mafia-like institution of Houston Methodist Hospital. The country club of hospitals within the Texas Medical Center, Houston Methodist wields immense financial and operational clout in Houston, with over $13 billion in assets in 2022. The hospital sponsors professional sports teams like the Houston Astros and contributes vast amounts of advertising money to the Houston Grand Opera, the

Houston Symphony, and the Houston Ballet. These donations come with heavy strings attached. I was writing exemptions for performing artists from all these groups who were mandated to take the COVID shots. The Houston Methodist brand saturates billboards, TV, and radio ads all over Houston—I'm assaulted with it multiple times a day.

As a small, insignificant presence in the grand scope of Methodist's vast domain, I questioned why they targeted me so aggressively. The logical answer was money, so I collaborated with attorneys Steve Mitby and Michael Barnhart, alongside investigative reporter Wayne Dolcefino, to sue the hospital for access to its financial records.

As a nonprofit, Houston Methodist enjoys tax exempt status from both the state of Texas and the IRS, and under provisions of the Texas Business Organization Code 22, Texas law requires them to allow members of the public to inspect its financial records. We requested but were denied the following information from the hospital:[8]

1. Financial documents detailing all revenue generated for the treatment and care of any COVID-19 patients at Methodist Hospital since March 1, 2019.
2. Financial documents, including contracts and ledgers, detailing any payments from any pharmaceutical company for the treatment of COVID-19 or use of specific drugs for COVID-19 patients since March 1, 2019, including vaccines.
3. Current compensation and identities of the top ten executives of Methodist Hospital.
4. Any additional 990 tax returns filed by Methodist after the 2019 tax return.
5. Documents detailing any bonuses provided to employees of Methodist hospital since March 1, 2019.

Our lawsuit hit a wall when Judge Lauren Reeder blocked discovery and granted summary judgment to the hospital. In her ruling, she stated, "The Court finds that the summary judgment record conclusively establishes that Defendants do not solicit public funds; rather, public gifts or donations are directed to The

5/27/2022 2:18:32 PM
Marilyn Burgess - District Clerk
Harris County
Envelope No: 64935180
By: NORTH, SHANNON
Filed: 5/27/2022 2:18:32 PM

Pgs-1

MODIX
7

No. 2022-02976

MARY T. BOWDEN, M.D. and DOLCEFINO COMMUNICATIONS, LLC d/b/a Dolcefino Consulting,	§	IN THE DISTRICT COURT OF
Plaintiffs,	§	
v.	§	HARRIS COUNTY, TEXAS
THE METHODIST HOSPITAL and TMH PHYSICIAN ORGANIZATION,	§	
Defendants.	§	234TH JUDICIAL DISTRICT

~~[PROPOSED]~~ ORDER GRANTING DEFENDANTS' MOTION FOR TRADITIONAL SUMMARY JUDGMENT

Having considered Defendants' Motion for Traditional Summary Judgment (the "Motion"), any responses and replies, other pleadings, papers, evidence on file, and the arguments of counsel, if any, the Court is of the opinion that the Motion should be GRANTED.

It is therefore ORDERED that Defendants' Motion for Traditional Summary Judgment is GRANTED; and

ORDERED that all of Plaintiffs' claims against Defendants are dismissed with prejudice.

The Court finds that the summary judgment record conclusively establishes that neither Defendant solicits funds from the public; instead, any public gifts or donations are provide[d] to a seperate entity, The Methodist Hospital Foundation, which in turn provides funding to Defendants.

This order disposes of all claims of Mary T. Bowden, M.D. and Dolcefino Communications, LLC d/b/a Dolcefino Consulting against Defendants The Methodist Hospital and TMH Physician Organization.

Accordingly, Defendants are exempt fro[m] the requirements of §22.353.

SIGNED on ________________, 2022.

Signed:
8/16/2022

Lauren Reeder

JUDGE PRESIDING

Methodist Hospital Foundation, a separate entity that funds Defendants. Thus, Defendants are exempt from §22.353 requirements."[9]

Judge Reeder's ruling protected the hospital's complex financial structure, which operates like a corporate shell game, dispersing donations and revenue across twenty-six affiliated corporations and foundations—a web too intricate to unravel without a judge's order and a forensic accountant. We appealed the summary judgment, but Justices Randy Wilson, Kevin Jewell, and Charles Spain of the Texas Fourteenth Court of Appeals dismissed our effort without a hearing, further guarding the hospital's financial secrets.

The loss did not dissuade me from trying again. I hired attorney Steven Biss to help me sue the hospital for defamation in response to their announcement to the world that I was "dangerous" and "harmful to the community." Harris County Judge Mike Engelhart dismissed my case (and interestingly blocked me on X without provocation). I appealed to the Texas Fourteenth Court of Appeals; Judges Frances Bourliot, Charles Spain, and Jerry Zimmerer ruled in favor of Methodist and ordered me to pay their attorney fees. I lost on a technicality—my affidavit was struck as it did not contain my date of birth or address. My attorney suffered a stroke soon after the appeal, and I believe his poor health led to the mistake.

This legal misstep cost me $166,514.28, with the potential for further expenses. When Biss, my attorney, became incapacitated, Dennis Postiglione, an experienced defamation lawyer from Austin, took over. I chose not to pursue the case further and asked if the settlement funds could be donated to a charity of Houston Methodist's choice, but they refused. I also entertained the possibility of reducing the fees in exchange for a non-disparagement clause, which they rejected. After six months of trying to get an answer from their unresponsive lawyers, Dennis finally was able to get their settlement terms in writing—none of which I disputed—and I promptly sent a check for the full amount along with the signed settlement agreement. However, after cashing the check, Houston Methodist reneged, complaining about something I posted about them on X. They now demand an additional $25,391.79 in interest. We are challenging this and seeking sanctions.

The financial and legal ordeal with Houston Methodist, compounded by their post-settlement demands, mirrors my ongoing struggle against the Texas Medical Board as I await their recommended disciplinary action. A generous donor is funding my appeal, led by attorney Robert Barnes, and I plan to sue the Board for violating my First Amendment and due process rights. With the help of attorney Ilya Feoktistov and along with three other physicians, I am also preparing a lawsuit against the Federation of State Medical Boards for similar constitutional infringements.

Our unexpected win over the FDA was a huge accomplishment and establishes crucial protections for the doctor-patient relationship against government overreach—but we still have a long way to go. The mRNA shots are still on the market, ivermectin is still difficult to access, and the vaccine-injured have been left behind. Trust in our healthcare system is at an all-time low, with only 17 percent of Americans feeling a great deal of confidence in the care they receive.[10] The government's response to the pandemic permanently stained the credibility of our public health agencies, and people no longer trust doctors like they once did.

The pandemic left our country with a large festering wound, and wounds of this magnitude do not heal on their own. Our only hope for repair is to correct the mistakes and demand accountability.

Attorney General Pam Bondi has yet to take action against the criminals of the pandemic, but in response to Biden's sweeping pardon of Fauci, seventeen state attorneys general, led by Alan Wilson of South Carolina, signed a letter to Speaker of the House Mike Johnson, asking for an investigation into Fauci's role in the pandemic response. Five of these states—Kansas, Texas, Utah,

Mississippi, and Louisiana—filed a suit against Pfizer for fraud, false advertising, and hiding adverse reactions.[11]

Rachel Rodriguez, founding attorney of Vires Law Group[12], has led a large effort to encourage county attorneys general to hold hospitals accountable for the inhumane treatment of COVID patients during the pandemic. Asserting crimes of capital murder, murder, manslaughter, trafficking of persons, racketeering, injury to and endangering children, the elderly, and the disabled, and unlawful restraint, Rachel's group has sent letters to twenty-two county attorneys general in Texas and several in two other states urging investigations. Of those, two district attorneys have taken interest and started investigations.

Meanwhile, a quiet but productive war has been waging in the civil courts. According to attorney and founder of Freedom Counsel network,[13] Warner Mendenhall, over twenty-five thousand COVID-related cases have been filed since the start of the pandemic. These cases are more successful than most people realize because many of them have settled privately; as of September 2025, Warner estimates the total payouts likely exceed $1 billion. While cases involving injuries from the COVID shots and hospital protocols are very challenging to win, litigation concerning violations of the False Claims Act hold more promise. With a statute of limitations of six years, the opportunity to file suits is still an option, and many whistleblowers have turned in employers who fraudulently filed claims under the Payroll Protection Program. Per Warner, a trillion dollars of pandemic fraud is waiting to be exposed.

One fraud case holds particular significance and, if successful, has the potential to topple the entire pandemic house of cards. Pfizer is being sued under the False Claims Act by whistleblower Brook Jackson, a research operations expert directly involved in Pfizer's mRNA trials. With two decades of experience, Brook accepted a new position as Regional Director of Operations with Ventavia

Research Group on September 8, 2020. Her primary responsibility was to oversee the conduct of Pfizer's Phase 3 COVID-19 mRNA trial at several locations in Texas. As operations director, Brook's job was to protect the rights, safety, and welfare of the people volunteering to be in the study and ensure the integrity of the information collected. Immediately she noticed problems, stating, "In the 20 years that I have been involved in clinical research, I have never seen a study conducted by an investigative site, managed by a contractor, or overseen by a pharmaceutical sponsor that scared me until then."[14]

Brook witnessed investigators glossing over informed consent, fabricating and falsifying data, failing to test ill patients, failing to keep clinicians blinded, and failing to report adverse events. She didn't wait, and after being there for only seventeen days, Brook reported her concerns to the FDA. Within hours, she was fired.

Three months later, Pfizer's mRNA shot received EUA approval. Brook looked at the study published in the *New England Journal of Medicine* used to justify the approval and knew the data from her site—encompassing 3 percent of the forty-four thousand subjects—wasn't excluded as it should have been. The consequences are potentially dire. To date, over 13.7 billion doses of the COVID shot have been given around the world to people who were told the product had been subjected to rigorous safety standards.

With the help of her attorneys, Warner Mendenhall and Robert Barnes, Brook filed a False Claims Act lawsuit against Pfizer in January 2021. Brook and her team asked the DOJ to assist, but they declined to get involved. As the case dragged on, Pfizer's attorneys were clearly getting outmaneuvered. In an unprecedented move, the DOJ parachuted in, intervening to try to stop the case from moving forward. Even with a new administration and Pam Bondi as our attorney general, the DOJ has continued to collude with Pfizer to push for dismissal, claiming the case goes against federal public health policies. The stakes are very high. If successful, Brook's case could bankrupt Pfizer and entirely dismantle the credibility of our public health system.

On a positive note, a lawsuit brought by the Department of Justice in 2023 against Dr. Kirk Moore was dismissed. Dr. Moore, a plastic surgeon in Utah, gave his patients a choice when the federal government would not. In response to the mandates, Dr. Moore offered saline instead of mRNA injections, saving over 1900 patients from harm. He charged no money for this service, only asking for recipients to make a charitable donation to a local medical freedom group. In January 2023, he and three associates were indicted by the US Attorney's Office on charges of conspiracy to defraud the United States, conversion of government property with aiding and abetting, and destruction of government property. If convicted on all counts, he would have faced up to thirty-five years in prison and a $125,000 judgment—but in mid-trial, US Attorney General Pam Bondi learned of what was happening and ordered the charges to be dropped.[15] Of the over one million physicians in the United States, only a small percentage of my colleagues had the courage to speak out and fight back during the pandemic. Facing forces larger than Goliath, our careers and personal lives have suffered tremendously—but as more information continues to surface, we are slowly being vindicated. By refusing to conform to institutional pressures, we faced (and still face) severe professional attacks—on our licenses, hospital privileges, and reputations. But rather than retreat, we went on offense; the attacks fueled our fire, prompting us to get louder and dedicate our limited free time to advocacy and exposing the many injustices brought forth by the pandemic. The crimes were nothing we'd ever encountered: the requirement to inject a gene therapy product with no long-term safety data, the lack of support to care for the vaccine-injured, and the trampling of our Constitutional rights to free speech and bodily autonomy. We suffered professionally to advocate for our patients, many of whom felt abandoned by a system prioritizing compliance over inquiry.

The last five years have been among the most challenging years I've ever experienced, yet they've shaped me profoundly. The toughest times often leave the deepest impact, and as an introvert who's faced lifelong criticism for being too quiet, I've found a voice I never knew I had. Though I've always held strong opinions, until the pandemic I mostly kept them to myself. When the pressure became overwhelming, I began sharing my thoughts in writing—through emails to my patients and on social media—and everything changed. I never imagined I'd end up giving speeches to large audiences or appearing on shows hosted by Tucker Carlson and Joe Rogan. I'm grateful to my adversaries for pushing me out of my shell. The hardship has set me free.

These battles have taken a personal toll. Practicing medicine has become more challenging. Media exposure means my patients often know more about me than I do about them, and every visit now involves discussions about current events. I've lost my privacy—a loss I can never reclaim—and the past five years have taken precious time away from my children. I'm scaling back my practice to recapture those moments before my children leave for college, but the steady stream of vaccine-injured patients strengthens my resolve to keep advocating for them.

The pandemic may be over, but the future of our country's healthcare system is still in chaos. As I write this, Secretary Kennedy is defending calls for his resignation, and states are breaking away from federal health guidelines, forming their own coalitions to set independent vaccination policies.

The chaos, though unsettling, is a positive sign of progress. In an ideal world, the villains suffer swift defeat, but we are not there yet. In the current post-COVID world, seemingly little progress has been made, but based on the volume of their shrieks, the medical establishment is starting to panic.

Pride, hatred, and injustice lead to inevitable defeat, while courage, faith, and standing on principle can overcome even the gravest threats. My advocacy persists in the hope that truth will eventually prevail. The triumph of good over evil resonates in my patients' resilience and my commitment to their care. Through unity and perseverance, we can protect the vulnerable and challenge systems that prioritize power over people. As tempting as it is to back away, the fight is far from over. Consider joining the effort if you haven't already.

Endnotes

Chapter 3

1 Richard Horton, "Vioxx, the Implosion of Merck, and Aftershocks at the FDA," *The Lancet* 364, no. 9450 (2004): 1995–96, https://doi.org/10.1016/s0140-6736(04)17523-5.

2 "Information for Healthcare Professionals: Fluoroquinolone Antimicrobial Drugs [Ciprofloxacin (Marketed as Cipro and Generic Ciprofloxacin), Ciprofloxacin Extended-Release (Marketed as Cipro XR and Proquin XR), Gemifloxacin (Marketed as Factive), Levofloxacin (Marketed as Levaquin), Moxifloxacin (Marketed as Avelox), Norfloxacin (Marketed as Noroxin), and Ofloxacin (Marketed as Floxin)]," U.S. Food and Drug Administration, archived October 22, 2016, at http://wayback.archive-it.org/7993/20161022101528/http://www.fda.gov/Drugs/DrugSafety/PostmarketDrugSafetyInformationforPatientsandProviders/ucm126085.htm.

3 "FDA Drug Safety Communication: FDA Requires Label Changes to Warn of Risk for Possibly Permanent Nerve Damage from Antibacterial Fluoroquinolone Drugs Taken by Mouth or by Injection," U.S. Department of Health and Human Services, archived October 22, 2016, at http://wayback.archive-it.org/7993/20161022101530/http://www.fda.gov/Drugs/DrugSafety/ucm365050.htm.

4 "FDA Drug Safety Communication: FDA Updates Warnings for Oral and Injectable Fluoroquinolone Antibiotics Due to Disabling Side Effects," U.S. Food and Drug Administration, effective May 12, 2016, https://www.fda.gov/drugs/drug-safety-and-availability/fda-drug-safety-

communication-fda-updates-warnings-oral-and-injectable-fluoroquinolone-antibiotics.

5 "FDA Warns about Increased Risk of Ruptures or Tears in the Aorta Blood Vessel with Fluoroquinolone Antibiotics in Certain Patients," U.S. Food and Drug Administration, last modified December 21, 2018, https://www.fda.gov/drugs/drug-safety-and-availability/fda-warns-about-increased-risk-ruptures-or-tears-aorta-blood-vessel-fluoroquinolone-antibiotics.

6 Marcel Yibirin, Diana De Oliveira, Roberto Valera, Andrea E Plitt, and Sophia Lutgen, "Adverse Effects Associated with Proton Pump Inhibitor Use," *Cureus* (2021), https://doi.org/10.7759/cureus.12759.

7 Nicholas S. Downing, Nilay D. Shah, Jenerius A. Aminawung, Alison M. Pease, Jean-David Zeitoun, Harlan M. Krumholz, and Joseph S. Ross, "Postmarket Safety Events among Novel Therapeutics Approved by the US Food and Drug Administration between 2001 and 2010," *JAMA* 317, no. 18 (2017): 1854, https://doi.org/10.1001/jama.2017.5150.

8 Karen E. Lasser, "Timing of New Black Box Warnings and Withdrawals for Prescription Medications," *JAMA* 287, no. 17 (2002): 2215, https://doi.org/10.1001/jama.287.17.2215.

9 Neal Nathanson and Alexander D. Langmuir, "The Cutter Incident: Poliomyelitis Following Formaldehyde-Inactivated Poliovirus Vaccination in the United States During the Spring of 1955: II. Relationship of Poliomyelitis to Cutter Vaccine," *American Journal of Epidemiology* 142, no. 2 (1995): 109–40, https://doi.org/10.1093/oxfordjournals.aje.a117611.

10 Regis A. Vilchez and Janet S. Butel, "Emergent Human Pathogen Simian Virus 40 and Its Role in Cancer," *Clinical Microbiology Reviews* 17, no. 3 (2004): 495–508, https://doi.org/10.1128/cmr.17.3.495-508.2004.

11 "Historical Vaccine Concerns," Centers for Disease Control and Prevention, effective July 31, 2024, https://www.cdc.gov/vaccine-safety/historical-concerns/index.html#:~:text=Simian%20Virus%2040%20(SV40):,vaccines%20were%20free%20of%20SV40.&text=No%20vaccines%20used%20today%20contain%20SV40%20virus.&text=Immunization%20Safety%20Review:%20SV40%20Contamination%20of%20Polio%20Vaccine%20and%20Cancer.

12 "Florida State Surgeon General Calls for Halt in the Use of COVID-19 mRNA Vaccines," Florida Health, effective January 3, 2024, https://www.floridahealth.gov/newsroom/2024/01/20240103-halt-use-covid19-mrna-vaccines.pr.html.

13 "Swine Flu 1976," Murphy Library, last modified December 4, 2025, 15:35 (UTC), https://libguides.uwlax.edu/govinfo/swine-flu-1976.

14 "Swine Flu Immunization Program of 1976," Gerald R. Ford Presidential Library and Museum, accessed December 4, 2025, https://www.fordlibrarymuseum.gov/digital-research-room/topic-guides/swine-flu-immunization-program-1976.

15 Gilles Delage, "Rotavirus Vaccine Withdrawal in the United States: The Role of Postmarketing Surveillance," *Canadian Journal of Infectious Diseases and Medical Microbiology* 11, no. 1 (2000): 10–12, https://doi.org/10.1155/2000/414396.

Chapter 4

1 "Governor Abbott Establishes Statewide Face Covering Requirement, Issues Proclamation to Limit Gatherings," Office of the Texas Governor | Greg Abbott, July 2, 2020, https://gov.texas.gov/news/post/governor-abbott-establishes-statewide-face-covering-requirement-issues-proclamation-to-limit-gatherings.

2 Holly Hansen, "New Study Supports West Texas Doctor's Early 'Silver Bullet' Covid-19 Treatment," *The Texan*, June 9, 2023, https://thetexan.news/issues/healthcare/new-study-supports-west-texas-doctor-s-early-silver-bullet-covid-19-treatment/article_f3a832aa-8de0-57aa-9b23-e10b25232594.html.

3 President Donald J. Trump, "Pres. Donald Trump: I'm taking hydroxychloroquine to prevent coronavirus infection," posted May 18, 2020, by CNBC Television, YouTube, 00:06:39, https://www.youtube.com/watch?v=7nkwE3didNo.

4 "Guidance Statements Re: Covid-19," Texas State Board of Pharmacy, effective May 15, 2020, https://www.pharmacy.texas.gov/files_pdf/TSBP-COVID-statement.pdf.

5 "Guidance Statements," Texas State Board of Pharmacy, 2020, https://www.pharmacy.texas.gov/files_pdf/TSBP-COVID-statement.pdf.

6 Denise M. Hinton, "Request for Emergency Use Authorization for Use of Chloroquine Phosphate or Hydroxychloroquine Sulfate Supplied from the Strategic National Stockpile for Treatment of 2019 Coronavirus Disease," U.S. Food and Drug Administration, effective March 28, 2020, https://www.washoecounty.gov/bcc/board_committees/2020/files/agendas/2020-04-00/Item10_ExhC_Final-FDA-Emergency-Use-Authorization-HydroxyChloroquine-and-ChloroquineLOA.pdf.

7 "Coronavirus (COVID-19) Update: FDA Revokes Emergency Use Authorization for Chloroquine and Hydroxychloroquine," U.S. Food and Drug Administration, effective June 15, 2020, https://www.fda.gov/news-events/press-announcements/coronavirus-covid-19-update-fda-revokes-emergency-use-authorization-chloroquine-and.

8 "TMA COVID–19 Task Force," Texas Medical Association, last modified July 13, 2021, https://ftp.texmed.org/Template.aspx?id=52913&terms=task+force%22+%5Ch.

9 Rob Stein, "The Latest Covid Vaccines Come with New FDA Limits," *NPR*, August 27, 2025, https://www.npr.org/sections/shots-health-news/2025/08/27/nx-s1-5515503/fda-covid-vaccines-restricted.

Chapter 5

1 David W. Feigal, Jr., "Approval Package," Center for Drug Evaluation and Research, effective November 22, 1996, https://www.accessdata.fda.gov/drugsatfda_docs/nda/96/050742ap.pdf.

2 "PRESS RELEASE: Joint Statement from TMB and TSBP Regarding Prescribed Drugs or Treatment for COVID-19," Texas State Board of Pharmacy, effective September 3, 2021, https://www.pharmacy.texas.gov/news/press-release/joint-statement-re-drugs-or-treatment-for-covid19.pdf.

3 Sabriya Rice, "In Texas, Pharmacists Can Refuse to Fill Your Prescriptions for Any Drug for Any Reason They Choose," The Dallas Morning News, June 25, 2018, https://www.dallasnews.com/business/health-care/2018/06/26/in-texas-pharmacists-can-refuse-to-fill-your-prescriptions-for-any-drug-for-any-reason-they-choose/.

4 Jacqueline Howard and Jen Christensen, "FDA Warns Against Using Anti-Parasitic Drug for Covid-19 After Reports of Hospitalizations," CNN Health, March 5, 2021, https://www.cnn.com/2021/03/05/health/ivermectin-covid-19-fda-statement-wellness#:~:text=CNN%20%E2%80%94,medications%2C%20such%20as%20blood%20thinners.

5 FOX19 Digital Staff, "FDA Dispels Myth About Animal Worm Drug as COVID Cure," FOX19 NOW, August 21, 2021, https://www.fox19.com/2021/08/21/seriously-yall-stop-it-fda-dispels-myth-about-ivermectin-covid-cure/.

6 Victor Nava, "Amazon 'Censored' COVID-19 Vaccine Books After 'Feeling Pressure' From Biden White House: Docs," *New York Post*, February 5, 2024, https://nypost.com/2024/02/05/news/amazon-censored-

covid-19-vaccine-books-after-feeling-pressure-from-biden-white-house-docs/.

7 "FACT SHEET: Biden Administration Announces Historic $10 Billion Investment to Expand Access to COVID-19 Vaccines and Build Vaccine Confidence in Hardest-Hit and Highest-Risk Communities," The White House, archived March 25, 2021, at https://bidenwhitehouse.archives.gov/briefing-room/statements-releases/2021/03/25/fact-sheet-biden-administration-announces-historic-10-billion-investment-to-expand-access-to-covid-19-vaccines-and-build-vaccine-confidence-in-hardest-hit-and-highest-risk-communities/.

8 "COVID-19 Community Corps: Social Media Launch Toolkit for HHS," COVID-19 Community Corps, April 1, 2021, https://www.cms.gov/files/document/socialmediatoolkithhs.pdf.

9 U.S. Department of Health and Human Services, "Over 15,000 COVID-19 Community Corps members, including individuals and organizations big and small," Facebook, November 1, 2021, https://www.facebook.com/HHS/videos/702084320768992/.

10 "2021 Triological Society 123rd Annual Meeting: Virtual Meeting at COSM," Triological Society, April 9–10, 2021, https://cdn.ymaws.com/triological.org/resource/resmgr/past_meetings/2021cosmprogramshort.pdf.

Chapter 6

1 Mary Talley Bowden, Christopher A. Church, Alexander G. Chiu, and Winston C. Vaughan, "Informed Consent in Functional Endoscopic Sinus Surgery: The Patient's Perspective," *Otolaryngology–Head and Neck Surgery* 131, no. 1 (2016): 126–32, https://doi.org/10.1016/j.otohns.2004.02.027.

2 Mary Talley Bowden, "Coercion is Not Consent," *Dangerous Misinformation,* November 12, 2023, https://drbowden.substack.com/p/coercion-is-not-consent?r=sezjh&utm_campaign=post&utm_medium=web&triedRedirect=true.

Chapter 7

1 Mary Talley Bowden, "No License for Disinformation," *Dangerous Misinformation,* June 19, 2022, https://drbowden.substack.com/p/no-license-for-disinformation.

2 Houston Methodist (@MethodistHosp), "Dr. Mary Bowden, who recently joined the medical staff at Houston Methodist Hospital, is using her social

media accounts to express her personal and political opinions about the COVID-19 vaccine and treatments," Twitter (now X), November 12, 2021, https://x.com/MethodistHosp/status/1459293932488208384.

Chapter 9

1 "Shots Heard Round The World Toolkit," Shots Heard Round The World, accessed December 5, 2025, https://vaccineresourcehub.org/sites/default/files/resources/files/Shots%2BHeard%2BToolkit.pdf

Chapter 10

1 "Federal Trade Commission v. U.S. Anesthesia Partners, Inc. et al.," O'Neill Institute Health Care Litigation Tracker, last modified November 14, 2025, https://litigationtracker.law.georgetown.edu/litigation/federal-trade-commission-v-u-s-anesthesia-partners-inc-et-al/#:~:text=Why%20this%20Matters,SEAL%20(Jul%2011%2C%20 2025).

Chapter 11

1 Purva Khare, Sara X. Edgecomb, Christine M. Hamadani, Eden E.L. Tanner, and Devika S Manickam, "Lipid Nanoparticle-Mediated Drug Delivery to the Brain," *Advanced Drug Delivery Reviews* 197 (2023): 114861, https://doi.org/10.1016/j.addr.2023.114861.

2 Hanna Nazeeh, Ari Heffes-Doon, Xinhua Lin, Claudia Manzano De Mejia, Bishoy Botros, Ellen Gurzenda, and Amrita Nayak, "Detection of Messenger RNA Covid-19 Vaccines in Human Breast Milk," *JAMA Pediatrics* 176, no. 12 (2022): 1268, https://doi.org/10.1001/jamapediatrics.2022.3581.

3 Pedro Morais, Hironori Adachi, and Yi-Tao Yu, "The Critical Contribution of Pseudouridine to mRNA COVID-19 Vaccines," *Frontiers in Cell and Developmental Biology* 9 (2021), https://doi.org/10.3389/fcell.2021.789427.

4 Bornali Bhattacharjee, Peiwen Lu, Valter Silva Monteiro, Alexandra Tabachnikova, Kexin Wang, William B. Hooper, Victoria Bastos, et al., Immunological and Antigenic Signatures Associated with Chronic Illnesses After Covid-19 Vaccination, *medRxiv* (2025), https://doi.org/10.1101/2025.02.18.25322379.

5 Sonia Ndeupen, Zhen Qin, Sonya Jacobsen, Aurélie Bouteau, Henri Estanbouli, and Botond Z. Igyártó, "The mRNA-LNP Platform's Lipid Nanoparticle Component Used in Preclinical Vaccine Studies Is Highly Inflammatory," *iScience* 24, no.12 (2021): 103479, https://doi.org/10.1016/j.isci.2021.103479.

6 Dzhigangir Faizullin, Yuliya Valiullina, Vadim Salnikov, and Yuriy Zuev, "Direct Interaction of Fibrinogen with Lipid Microparticles Modulates Clotting Kinetics and Clot Structure," *Nanomedicine: Nanotechnology, Biology and Medicine* 23 (2020): 102098, https://doi.org/10.1016/j.nano.2019.102098.

7 Stéphanie Andrade, Joana A. Loureiro, Santiago Ramirez, Celso S. Catumbela, Claudio Soto, Rodrigo Morales, and Maria Carmo Pereira, "Multi-Dose Intravenous Administration of Neutral and Cationic Liposomes in Mice: An Extensive Toxicity Study," *Pharmaceuticals* 15, no. 6 (2022): 761, https://doi.org/10.3390/ph15060761.

8 William M. Pardridge, "Brain Gene Therapy with Trojan Horse Lipid Nanoparticles," *Trends in Molecular Medicine* 29, no. 5 (2023): 343–53, https://doi.org/10.1016/j.molmed.2023.02.004.

9 Emanuele Nappi, Francesca Racca, Alessandra Piona, Maria Messina, Sebastian Ferri, Donatella Lamacchia, Giuseppe Cataldo, et al., "Polyethylene Glycol and Polysorbate 80 Skin Tests in the Context of an Allergic Risk Assessment for Hypersensitivity Reactions to Anti-SARS-Cov-2 Mrna Vaccines," *Vaccines* 11, no. 5 (2023): 915, https://doi.org/10.3390/vaccines11050915.

10 Michael Capuzzo, "Top Doctors at Summit Today: 'Healthy Children Shall Not Be Subject to Forced Vaccination,'" *RESCUE with Michael Capuzzo,* November 6, 2021, https://rescue.substack.com/p/top-doctors-at-summit-today-healthy.

11 Capuzzo, "Top Doctors at Summit Today," 2021, https://rescue.substack.com/p/top-doctors-at-summit-today-healthy.

12 "US Coronavirus Vaccine Tracker," USA FACTS, last modified May 10, 2025, https://usafacts.org/visualizations/covid-vaccine-tracker-states/.

13 Roy Maurer, "Biden Orders Vaccination Mandates for Larger Employers, Federal Workforce," *SHRM,* September 9, 2021, https://www.shrm.org/topics-tools/news/talent-acquisition/biden-orders-vaccination-mandates-larger-employers-federal-workforce.

14 Ross Lazarus, "Electronic Support for Public Health–Vaccine Adverse Event Reporting System (ESP:VAERS)," *Grant Final Report,* R18 HS 017045 (2010), https://digital.ahrq.gov/sites/default/files/docs/publication/r18hs017045-lazarus-final-report-2011.pdf.

15 Deborah Conrad, "Seeking Justice Support our Qui Tam Whistleblower," GiveSendGo, accessed December 5, 2025, https://www.givesendgo.com/GCBG5.

16 "I-Recover Post-Vaccine Treatment Guide," Independent Medical Alliance, accessed December 5, 2025, https://imahealth.org/protocol/i-recover-post-vaccine-treatment/.

17 "Table 4. CICP Claims Compensated (Fiscal Years 2010 – 2025)," Health Resources and Services Administration, last modified November 1, 2025, https://www.hrsa.gov/cicp/cicp-data/table-4.

Chapter 12

1 "Confronting Health Misinformation: The U.S. Surgeon General's Advisory on Building a Healthy Information Environment," Surgeon General of the United States, 2021, https://www.hhs.gov/sites/default/files/surgeon-general-misinformation-advisory.pdf.

2 "Joint Statement on Dissemination of Misinformation," American Board of Internal Medicine, September 9, 2021, https://www.abim.org/media/press-releases/joint-statement-on-dissemination-of-misinformation/.

3 "Klobuchar, Luján Urge Tech CEOs to Take Action Against 'Disinformation Dozen,' Combat Coronavirus Vaccine Disinformation," United States Senator Amy Klobuchar, April 19, 2021, https://www.klobuchar.senate.gov/public/index.cfm/2021/4/klobuchar-luj-n-urge-tech-ceos-to-take-action-against-disinformation-dozen-combat-coronavirus-vaccine-disinformation.

4 Taylor Hatmaker, "Democratic Bill Would Suspend Section 230 Protections When Social Networks Boost Anti-Vax Conspiracies," TechCrunch, July 22, 2021, https://techcrunch.com/2021/07/22/section-230-health-misinformation-act/.

5 Shannon N. Glueck, letter to Humayun J. Chaudhry, December 13, 2021, https://content.govdelivery.com/attachments/WIDHS/2021/12/22/file_attachments/2030302/Ivermectin%20Letter%20to%20FSMB%20Final%20%281%29.pdf?fbclid=IwAR0aWt7v2hYCwGc2gJQ9DYk2SC-c6Zh08NYuTXaQmS5J4XYEE88qYJPe8kA8.

6 CNN, "Biden Says Platforms Like Facebook Are 'Killing People; with COVID-19 Misinformation," CTV News, July 16, 2021, https://www.ctvnews.ca/lifestyle/article/biden-says-platforms-like-facebook-are-killing-people-with-covid-19-misinformation/.

7 Leia Idliby, "Surgeon General Blames Big Tech for Letting Covid Misinformation Run Rampant: This 'Poison' Poses an 'Imminent and Insidious Threat,'" Mediaite, July 15, 2021, https://www.mediaite.com/media/tv/surgeon-general-blames-big-tech-for-letting-covid-misinformation-run-rampant-this-poison-poses-an-imminent-and-insidious-threat/.

8 Donie O'Sullivan, "Twitter Is No Longer Enforcing Its Covid Misinformation Policy," CNN Business, November 29, 2022, https://www.cnn.com/2022/11/29/tech/twitter-covid-misinformation-policy.

9 Mary Talley Bowden MD (@MaryBowdenMD), "Lawyer up @twitter and @cdc. @America1stLegal obtains emails between CDC director of digital media Carol Crawford and @Twitter execs on how to suppress free speech. Examples in thread," Twitter (now X), July 28, 2022, https://x.com/MaryBowdenMD/status/1552701966983348224.

Chapter 15

1 Vinay Prasad and Martin A. Makary, "An Evidence-Based Approach to Covid-19 Vaccination," *New England Journal of Medicine* 392, no. 24 (2025): 2484–86, https://doi.org/10.1056/nejmsb2506929.

2 "Cardiac Complications After SARS-CoV-2 Infection and mRNA COVID-19 Vaccination — PCORnet, United States, January 2021–January 2022," CDC Morbidity and Mortality Weekly Report (*MMWR*), April 8, 2022, https://www.cdc.gov/mmwr/volumes/71/wr/mm7114e1.htm.

3 "COVID-19 VaST Work Group Report – May 17, 2021," National Center for Immunization and Respiratory Diseases, archived June 10, 2024, at https://archive.cdc.gov/www_cdc_gov/vaccines/acip/work-groups-vast/report-2021-05-17.html.

4 Dror Mevorach, Emilia Anis, Noa Cedar, Michal Bromberg, Eric J. Haas, Eyal Nadir, Sharon Olsha-Castell, et al., "Myocarditis After BNT162b2 Mrna Vaccine Against Covid-19 in Israel," *New England Journal of Medicine* 385, no. 23 (2021): 2140–49, https://doi.org/10.1056/nejmoa2109730.

5 Supriya S. Jain, Steven A. Anderson, Jeremy M. Steele, Hunter C. Wilson, Juan Carlos Muniz, Jonathan H. Soslow, Rebecca S. Beroukhim, et al., "Cardiac Manifestations and Outcomes of COVID-19 Vaccine-Associated Myocarditis in the Young in the USA: Longitudinal Results from the Myocarditis after COVID Vaccination (Maciv) Multicenter Study," *eClinicalMedicine* 76 (2024): 102809, https://doi.org/10.1016/j.eclinm.2024.102809.

6 Panagis Polykretis and Peter A. McCullough, "Rational Harm-Benefit Assessments by Age Group Are Required for Continued Covid-19 Vaccination," *Scandinavian Journal of Immunology* 98, no. 1 (2023), https://doi.org/10.1111/sji.13242.

7 Nathaniel M. Mead, "Myocarditis After SARS-COV-2 Infection and COVID-19 Vaccination: Epidemiology, Outcomes, and New Perspectives," *International Journal of Cardiovascular Research & Innovation* (2025), https://doi.org/10.61577/ijcri.2025.100001.

8 Grady Means, "American 'Genocide': Monetizing the Great Reset," *The Hill*, February 22, 2023, https://thehill.com/opinion/healthcare/3865837-american-genocide-monetizing-the-great-reset/.

9 Jamie Ducharme, "A Major Drug Company Now Has Access to 23andMe's Genetic Data. Should You Be Concerned?" *Time*, July 26, 2018, https://time.com/5349896/23andme-glaxo-smith-kline/.

Chapter 16

1 Hoyt Sze and Madeline Townsley, "Potential False Claims Act Liability for Providers of Gender-Affirming Care for Minors," *White Collar and Government Enforcement Blog*, July 30, 2025, https://www.whitecollarlawblog.com/2025/07/potential-false-claims-act-liability-for-providers-of-gender-affirming-care-for-minors/#:~:text=Specifically%2C%20the%20complaints%20allege%20the,not%20cover%20gender%2Daffirming%20care.

2 John Egan, "Houston Boasts Massive Population Growth Among Major U.S. Metros From 2010 to 2020," *innovationmap*, August 16, 2021, https://houston.innovationmap.com/houston-census-growth-ranking-of-largest-metro-areas-2654682995.html.

3 "Census Data Shows in 1st Full Year of Pandemic, Residents Left Big Metros Outside of Texas," abc13 Eyewitness News, March 24, 2022, https://abc13.com/post/california-population-californians-moving-to-texas-houston-us-census-bureau/11678209/.

4 "Texas High Growth Report Summery 2023: Predicting High-Demand Occupations Through 2030," Texas Workforce Commission, accessed December 5, 2025, https://lmi.twc.texas.gov/shared/PDFs/High-Growth-Annual-Report-Final-Review-summary.pdf.

5 "Texas Hiring Trends 2025: What Industries Are Growing Fastest," Burnett Specialists, August 12, 2025, https://burnettspecialists.com/blog/texas-hiring-trends-2025-what-industries-are-growing-fastest/#:~:text=1.,Accounting%2C%20Finance%20&%20Payroll%20Services.

6 "About Us," Texas Medical Center, accessed December 5, 2025, https://www.tmc.edu/about-tmc/.

7 "Gross Domestic Product: Health Care and Social Assistance (62) in Texas," FRED, last modified September 26, 2025, https://fred.stlouisfed.org/series/TXHLTHSOCASSNQGSP#:~:text=Data%20%3E%20States%20%3E%20Texas-,Gross%20Domestic%20Product:%20Health%20Care%20and%20Social%20Assistance%20(62),Release%20Date:%20Sep%2026%2C%202025.

8 Sean Price, "Texas Physician Growth Remains Strong, But Robust Recruitment Still Needed," *Texas Medical Association*, August 22, 2022, https://www.texmed.org/Template.aspx?id=60261#:~:text=Texas%20has%20made%20great%20strides,Patient%20Access%2C%20which%20includes%20TMA.

9 "Medical Residency in Texas," Residency Programs List, accessed December 5, 2025, https://www.residencyprogramslist.com/in-texas.

10 "The Graduate Medical Education Report: An Assessment of Opportunities for Graduates of Texas Medical Schools to Enter Residency Programs in Texas," Texas Higher Education Coordinating Board, October 2024, https://reportcenter.highered.texas.gov/reports/legislative/the-graduate-medical-education-report-an-assessment-of-opportunities-for-graduates-of-texas-medical-schools-to-enter-residency-programs-in-texas-2024/.

11 "Health Professionals PACs Contributions to Candidates, 2023-2024," OpenSecrets, last modified February 6, 2025, https://www.opensecrets.org/political-action-committees-pacs/industry-detail/H01/2024.

12 "Texas Medical Assn PAC Contributions to Federal Candidates," OpenSecrets, last modified February 6, 2025, https://www.opensecrets.org/political-action-committees-pacs/texas-medical-assn/C00001214/candidate-recipients/2024.

13 "Texas Medical Association Foundation," ProPublica, last modified November 19, 2025, https://projects.propublica.org/nonprofits/organizations/746073346/202303119349303640/full.

14 https://www.texmed.org/Template.aspx?id=42803&terms=135.013*

15 https://www.texmed.org/Template.aspx?id=57348&terms=135.029*

16 Greg Abbott, et al., v. Jane Doe, et al., 3rd App. Ct. TX (September 7, 2022), https://www.aclu.org/wp-content/uploads/legal-documents/2022.09.07_Amicus_Brief_of_Texas_Medical_Association_ISO_Appellees.pdf.

17 Mary Talley Bowden MD (@MaryBowdenMD), "I had no idea Houston's @TexasChildrens hospital touted itself as the preeminent, top-tier

transgender medical program in the US," Twitter (now X), March 10, 2022, https://x.com/MaryBowdenMD/status/1502106149222596632.

18 Greg Abbott, et al. (September 7, 2022), https://www.aclu.org/wp-content/uploads/legal-documents/2022.09.07_Amicus_Brief_of_Texas_Medical_Association_ISO_Appellees.pdf.

19 "Lambda Legal, A Nonprofit Supporting LGBTQ Rights, Exceeded Fundraising Goal by $105 Million," *The Chronicle of Philanthropy*, https://www.philanthropy.com/news/lambda-legal-a-nonprofit-supporting-lgbtq-rights-exceeded-fundraising-goal-by-105m/.

20 "Loe v. Texas," American Civil Liberties Union, last modified March 11, 2025, https://www.aclu.org/cases/loe-v-texas.

21 "Act 626 of 2021," Encyclopedia of Arkansas, last modified November 23, 2025, https://encyclopediaofarkansas.net/entries/act-626-of-2021-15789/.

22 Patrick McDaid, "Leading Through Change: TMA's Impact on Public Health Evident at State Level," *Texas Medicine June* 2024, last modified June 4, 2024, https://www.texmed.org/TexasMedicineDetail.aspx?Pageid=46106&id=64280.

23 "Dr. John Hellerstedt Receives THA Trustee Award for Public Health Leadership Throughout the COVID-19 Pandemic," Texas Hospital Association, accessed December 5, 2025, https://www.tha.org/news-publications/newsroom/dr-john-hellerstedt-receives-tha-trustee-award-for-public-health-leadership-throughout-the-covid-19-pandemic/#:~:text=%E2%80%9CTexas%20is%20stronger%20and%20more,The%20earliest%20days%20of%20Dr.

24 McDaid, "Leading Through Change," 2024, https://www.texmed.org/TexasMedicineDetail.aspx?Pageid=46106&id=64280.

25 McDaid, "Leading Through Change," 2024, https://www.texmed.org/TexasMedicineDetail.aspx?Pageid=46106&id=64280.

Chapter 17

1 Charles-Hervé Vacheron, Alain Lepape, Anne Savey, Anaïs Machut, Jean Francois Timsit, Philippe Vanhems, Quoc Viet Le, et al., "Increased Incidence of Ventilator-Acquired Pneumonia in Coronavirus Disease 2019 Patients: A Multicentric Cohort Study*," *Critical Care Medicine* 50, no. 3 (2022): 449–59, https://doi.org/10.1097/ccm.0000000000005297.

2 Originally available at this source, though the article has since been removed. Rasmussen TS, et al., "Nutritional Challenges In Hospitalized

Patients During The COVID-19 Pandemic: A Multicenter Study," *J Clin Nurs.* 31, no. 19–20 (2022): 2831–2840.

3 Cindy H. Liu, Emily Zhang, Ga Tin Wong, Sunah Hyun, and Hyeouk "Chris" Hahm, "Factors Associated with Depression, Anxiety, and PTSD Symptomatology During the COVID-19 Pandemic: Clinical Implications for U.S. Young Adult Mental Health," *Psychiatry Research* 290 (2020): 113172, https://doi.org/10.1016/j.psychres.2020.113172.

4 Terry E. Goldberg, Chen Chen, Yuanjia Wang, Eunice Jung, Antoinette Swanson, Caleb Ing, Paul S. Garcia, Robert A. Whittington, and Vivek Moitra, "Association of Delirium with Long-Term Cognitive Decline," *JAMA Neurology* 77, no. 11 (2020): 1373, https://doi.org/10.1001/jamaneurol.2020.2273.

5 Lixue Huang, Qun Yao, Xiaoying Gu, Qiongya Wang, Lili Ren, Yeming Wang, Ping Hu, et al., "1-Year Outcomes in Hospital Survivors with Covid-19: A Longitudinal Cohort Study," *The Lancet* 398, no. 10302 (2021): 747–58, https://doi.org/10.1016/s0140-6736(21)01755-4.

6 Lauren J. Breen, Sherman A. Lee, and Robert A. Neimeyer, "Psychological Risk Factors of Functional Impairment After COVID-19 Deaths," *Journal of Pain and Symptom Management* 61, no. 4 (2021), https://doi.org/10.1016/j.jpainsymman.2021.01.006.

7 Originally available at this source, though the article has since been removed. M. C. Eisma, A. Tamminga, G. E. Smid, P.A. Boelen, "Grief and Post-Traumatic Stress Following Bereavement During the COVID-19 Pandemic: A Meta-Analysis," *Front Psychiatry* 13 (2022): 846619.

8 Holly G. Prigerson and Paul K. Maciejewski, "Prolonged Grief Disorder," *The Lancet Psychiatry* 9, no. 9 (2022): 696, https://doi.org/10.1016/s2215-0366(22)00263-2.

9 Originally available at this source, though the article has since been removed. C. Campos-Castillo, J. L. Woodworth, B. L. Kaysen, et al., "How Do Family Members' Experiences with Care Shape Patient Trust in Medical Care?" *Soc Sci Med.* 287 (2021): 114313.

10 Jonathan Grein, Norio Ohmagari, Daniel Shin, George Diaz, Erika Asperges, Antonella Castagna, Torsten Feldt, et al., "Compassionate Use of Remdesivir for Patients with Severe COVID-19," *New England Journal of Medicine* 382, no. 24 (2020): 2327–36, https://doi.org/10.1056/nejmoa2007016.

11 John H. Beigel, Kay M. Tomashek, Lori E. Dodd, Aneesh K. Mehta, Barry S. Zingman, Andre C. Kalil, Elizabeth Hohmann, et al., "Remdesivir for the Treatment of Covid-19 — Final Report," *New England Journal of Medicine* 383, no. 19 (2020): 1813–26, https://doi.org/10.1056/nejmoa2007764.

12 WHO Solidarity Trial Consortium, "Repurposed Antiviral Drugs for Covid-19 — Interim Who Solidarity Trial Results," *New England Journal of Medicine* 384, no. 6 (2020): 497–511, https://doi.org/10.1056/nejmoa2023184.

13 Originally available at this source, though the article has since been removed. S. E. Tanni, a. Silvinato, I. Floriano, H. A. Bacha, A. N. Barbosa, W. M. Bernardo, "Use of Remdesivir in Patients with COVID-19: A Systematic Review and Meta-Analysis," *J. Bras Pneumol* 48, no. 1 (2022): e20210393.

14 Originally available at this source, though the article has since been removed. G. G. Pattullo, et al., "Opioid Therapy for Dyspnea in Patients with Advanced Pulmonary Disease: Balancing Benefits and Risks," *J. Pain Symptom Manage* 61, no. 4 (2021): 848–857.

15 Daniel Schorn, "Was It Murder?" *60 Minutes CBS News*, September 21, 2006, https://www.cbsnews.com/news/was-it-murder/.

16 Mary Talley Bowden MD (@MaryBowdenMD), "'When you go into a hospital, you sign your rights away.' Powerful words from @MendenhallFirm following unjust verdict in trial against Ascension Health," Twitter (now X), June 22, 2025, https://x.com/MaryBowdenMD/status/1936924177413329391.

Chapter 18

1 "Bylaws of The Federation of State Medical Boards Research and Education Foundation," FSMB Foundation, accessed December 5, 2025, https://www.fsmb.org/siteassets/foundation/foundation-bylaws.pdf.

2 "Federation of State Medical Boards of the United States Inc," ProPublica, last modified November 19, 2025, https://projects.propublica.org/nonprofits/organizations/751092490?utm_source=chatgpt.com%22%20\t%20%22_new%22.

3 "Report of the FSMB Ethics and Professionalism Committee: Professional Expectations Regarding Medical Misinformation and Disinformation," FSMB Board of Directors, April 2022, https://www.fsmb.org/siteassets/communications/tab-h2-brd-rpt-22-1-misinformation.pdf.

4 "Disinformation and Public Health," World Health Organization, effective February 6, 2024, https://www.who.int/news-room/questions-and-answers/item/disinformation-and-public-health#:~:text=What%20are%20misinformation%20and%20disinformation,and%20law%20enforcement%2C%20among%20others.

5 "Professional Expectations Regarding Medical Misinformation and Disinformation," FSMB House of Delegates, April 2022, https://www.fsmb.org/siteassets/advocacy/policies/ethics-committee-report-misinformation-april-2022-final.pdf.

6 Rachel L. Levine, "The government scrubbed this from the internet....," posted September 5, 2025, by Dr. Mary Talley Bowden, YouTube, 00:39:21, https://www.youtube.com/watch?v=yELrNkG0YTg.

7 "House of Delegates Annual Business Meeting," FSMB House of Delegates, April 2022, https://fsmbus.imiscloud.com/common/Uploaded%20files/AM%202022/2022%20HOD%20Book%20FINAL.pdf.

Chapter 19

1 "The MAHA Report," President Donald J. Trump, accessed December 5, 2025, https://www.whitehouse.gov/wp-content/uploads/2025/05/MAHA-Report-The-White-House.pdf.

2 The MAHA Report," The White House, accessed December 5, 2025, https://www.whitehouse.gov/maha/.

3 "COVID-19 Vaccination Implementation," National Center for Immunization and Respiratory Diseases, September 19, 2025, https://www.cdc.gov/acip/downloads/slides-2025-09-18-19/03-srinivasan-covid-508.pdf.

4 "mRESVIA FDA Approval History," Drugs.com, last modified June 13, 2025, https://www.drugs.com/history/mresvia.html.

5 Maryanne Demasi, "EXCLUSIVE: Did the CDC Mislead Its Advisers on the RSV Antibody for Babies?" Maryanne Demasi, reports, August 17, 2025, https://blog.maryannedemasi.com/p/exclusive-did-the-cdc-mislead-its?utm_medium=ios.

6 "Interim Clinical Considerations for Use of COVID-19 Vaccines in the United States," CDC, November 4, 2025, https://www.cdc.gov/covid/hcp/vaccine-considerations/index.html.

7 Sony Salzman, Will McDuffie, and Dr. Jade Cobern, "CDC Panel Abandons COVID Vaccine Recommendation, Saying It's a Personal Choice," abc News, September 19, 2025, https://abcnews.go.com/Health/cdc-hepatitis-bvaccine-vote-delayed-parents/story?id=125731004.

8 https://substack.com/@mdbreathe/p-60450396

9 https://www.hcdistrictclerk.com/Edocs/Public/CaseDetails.aspx?Get=UJGZFZxtS1IMj5aCfh1D7aX7+jt9zHaCS7xEJ30nbPvP-Wau%2fpwzPDrSxCZIABjqfH3CkYMGjJkVx3ZD2xXz3hXAQK6O-lOEF0JoZ4i4G1RHY%3d

10 Jane Sarasohn-Kahn, "Trust in Institutions Among Americans: Small Biz, the Military and Police More than the Medical System," Health Populi, July 15, 2024, https://www.healthpopuli.com/2024/07/15/trust-in-institutions-among-americans-small-biz-the-military-and-policy-more-than-the-medical-system/.

11 Tuhin Das Mahapatra, "These Five US States Are Suing Pfizer Over COVID-19 Vaccine Safety, Robert F Kennedy Jr Backs It," Hindustan Times, June 26, 2024, https://www.hindustantimes.com/world-news/us-news/robert-f-kennedy-jr-backs-lawsuits-against-pfizer-over-covid-19-vaccine-safety-the-tide-is-turning-101719371877572.html.

12 Home Page, Vires Law Group, accessed December 5, 2025, https://vireslaw.group/.

13 "Our Mission," Freedom Council, accessed December 5, 2025, https://freedomcounsel.org/.

14 "Who I Am," I Am Brook Jackson, accessed December 5, 2025, https://www.iambrookjackson.com/.

15 Maia Davies, "US Drops Charges Against Doctor Accused of Destroying Covid Vaccines," BBC, July 13, 2025, https://www.bbc.com/news/articles/cy0w1p0wq87o.